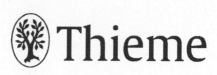

Textbook of Radiology for Cochlear Implants

Editor-in-Chief

Mohnish Grover, MS (ENT), FACS, PGDHHM
Professor
Department of Otorhinolaryngology
Additional Superintendent
SMS Medical College and Hospital
Jaipur, Rajasthan, India

Associate Editors

Gaurav Gupta
Professor
Department of Otorhinolaryngology
SP Medical College
Bikaner, Rajasthan, India

C Preetam
Professor
Department of Otorhinolaryngology
All India Institute of Medical Sciences
Bhubaneswar, Orissa, India

Thieme
Delhi • Stuttgart • New York • Rio de Janeiro

Publishing Director: Ritu Sharma
Senior Development Editor: Dr Gurvinder Kaur
Director-Editorial Services: Rachna Sinha
Project Manager: Aishwarya Panday
Vice President, Sales and Marketing: Arun Kumar Majji
Managing Director & CEO: Ajit Kohli

Thieme Medical and Scientific Publishers Private
Limited.
A - 12, Second Floor, Sector - 2, Noida - 201 301,
Uttar Pradesh, India, +911204556600
Email: customerservice@thieme.in
www.thieme.in

Cover design: © Thieme
Cover image source: © Thieme

Page make-up by RECTO Graphics, India

Printed in India

5 4 3 2 1

ISBN (print): 978-93-92819-26-1
eISBN (PDF): 978-93-92819-27-8
eISBN (epub): 978-93-92819-29-2

Contents

Foreword

In this age of the Internet, we are continuously and hopelessly drowning in a sea of information, forever filtering the useful from the useless, but not always knowing the difference. We increasingly rely on a Google search to answer every query—a search of over 40 zettabytes of information, with each zettabyte being a trillion gigabytes—that not surprisingly results in an equally large data dump, requiring time and energy to sift through to find the most meaningful facts and figures. With the publication of this textbook on cochlear implant radiology by Professor Mohnish Grover and his team, we now have a comprehensive resource to answer any conceivable question regarding imaging for cochlear implantation. Using his broad medical and surgical experience in cochlear implantation, as well as a deep understanding and encyclopedic knowledge of inner ear development, Professor Grover reviews the radiology of external, middle, and inner ear, central pathologies, as well as normal and abnormal anatomy, and their relevance for cochlear implantation. In a world filled with information noise, this book is a gift to all of us—Professor Grover has done the work for us and we no longer have to do mindless searches. This book is destined to be a classic!

Anil K. Lalwani, MD
Professor and Vice Chair for Research
Co-Director, Columbia Cochlear Implant Center
Department of Otolaryngology—Head & Neck Surgery
Associate Dean for Student Research
Columbia Vagelos College of Physicians and Surgeons
New York City, New York, USA

Preface

Over the past 17 years, as I treaded through the world of cochlear implants, I realized three things: First, the unknown inner ear anatomy has several intricacies than the well-explored complex middle ear. Second, the field of cochlear implants is one of the most rapidly changing areas of medical science. Last but probably the most important, reading and analyzing radiology is essential, especially because of the constant technological advances in the field and clinical significance of even the minutest details. During this period, I realized the need of a book which dealt with radiology related to cochlear implants in a detailed yet simplistic manner. This motivated me to write one. Authoring this book has been a wonderful learning experience for me too.

This book carries the essence of everything that I have learnt about application of radiology in the field of cochlear implants. I believe it will be an informative read for surgeons, radiologists, audiologists, and speech language pathologists who want to work in the field of cochlear implants. The images in the text with color-coded labeling will make the read interesting and easy to understand. Starting from basics, the chapters progress from normal radiology of temporal bones to more advanced topics such as malformations, ossification, and other inner ear and central pathologies. At the end there is a checklist which I recommend to be used during reporting of radiology for cochlear implants.

I thanks the coeditors Dr. C. Preetam and Dr. Gaurav Gupta for their help, and others who have contributed to this book in various ways. I thank my teachers at AIIMS, New Delhi, and PGIMER, Chandigarh, who have made me what I am in this field. I also gratefully acknowledge my colleagues at SMS Medical College, Jaipur, India (especially the ENT and Radiology Department) and families of cochlear implant recipients. I thank the publishing and editorial staff of Thieme, who guided the whole project from the first draft to finished textbook. Last but not the least, I thank my parents, my wife Shruti, and my children Nehal and Nibhish for bearing with me while I was busy writing this book.

Mohnish Grover, MS (ENT), FACS, PGDHHM

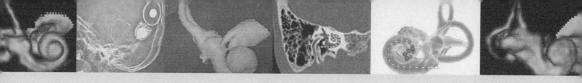

Chapter 1

Basics of CT and MRI

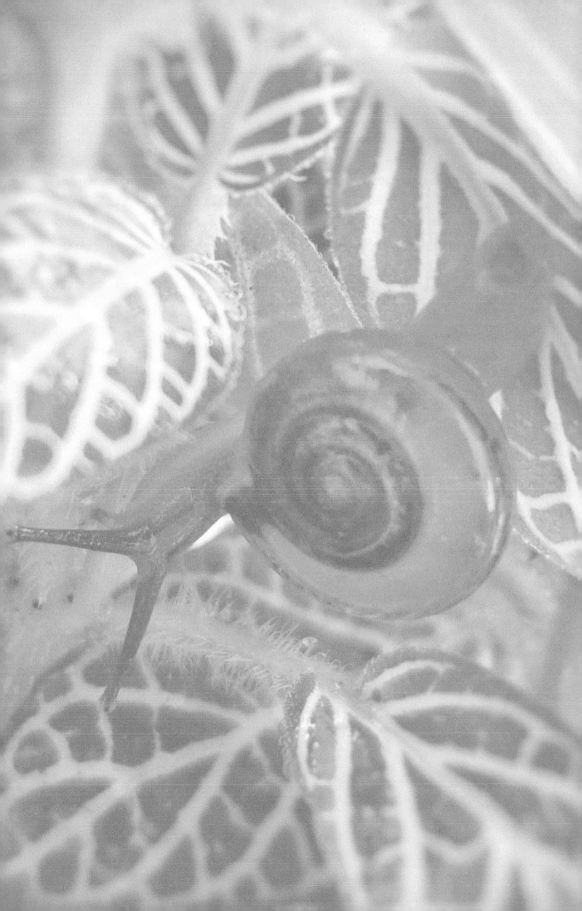

1 Basics of CT and MRI

Introduction

Cochlear implant (CI) has been a medical–engineering hybrid boon to patients with hearing loss. The results of CI are majorly dependent on candidacy, and radiology forms an imperative part of this work-up. Radiology not only helps in deciding the fitness for surgery but also is important as a roadmap for surgery. This helps in analyzing the possible risks during surgery and thereby helps the surgeon to counsel the patient in a better and honest manner.

High-resolution computed tomography (HRCT) of the temporal bone and magnetic resonance imaging (MRI) of the brain and temporal bone form the pillars of radiological evaluation for cochlear implant.[1] Few centers across the world have started shifting toward either one of them;[2,3] however, at least for people who are starting with cochlear implantation, the authors would recommend that both these investigations should be done in the best interest of the patient.

With the advent of technology, CT and MRI have become more accessible and economic. Also, better techniques have made them more useful and safe. These advantages have added safety to various neuro-otological surgeries.

It goes without saying that there should be a close collaboration between the surgeon and the radiologist so that the technology can be put to the best use. Surgeons often complain that radiologists do not provide correct sections or sequences or the reporting is suboptimal. At the same time, majority of radiologists feel that the surgeons do not provide adequate clinical details and the things required in reporting. The authors have found in their practice that good communication should be able to resolve majority of these issues.

Computed Tomography

Planes

To define the axis of various planes used in radiology it is imperative to define a true horizontal or transverse plane. To avoid any ambiguity, Reid's baseline was defined. Initially, it was defined as a line drawn from the inferior orbital margin to the center of the orifice of the external auditory canal.[4] However, in 1962, World Federation of Radiology changed the second point to the upper margin of the external auditory meatus.[4,5] This is used as zero plane in radiology. With the head upright, this plane corresponds to approximately 7 degrees nose up with respect to the horizontal plane which we usually perceive.

The most important cut for CI radiology is the axial plane (like for other temporal bone pathologies). Axial plane in the HRCT of the temporal bone is not true horizontal. It is at 30 degrees to Reid's baseline. Therefore, the axial plane is in the plane of the lateral semicircular canal. Coronal plane is perpendicular to the axial plane and therefore at 30 degrees to true vertical. **Fig. 1.1** shows these planes in pictographic form. This is a major difference from the radiology of other areas in the head and neck such as CT of paranasal sinuses where axial and coronal planes are in plane of true horizontal and vertical, respectively.

Hounsfield Units

Hounsfield unit (HU) is also called the "CT number." It is a relative quantitative measurement of radiodensity used in the interpretation of CT images.[6] HU is named after Sir Godfrey Hounsfield, a recipient of Nobel Prize in Physiology or Medicine in 1979 for the invention of CT.[7] A CT image is made up of a large number of pixels of varying gray scale. The level of gray scale is dependent on the density of the material or the linear absorption/ attenuation coefficient of radiation within a tissue. The physical density of tissue is proportional to the absorption/attenuation of the X-ray beam.[8] HU is calculated based on a linear transformation of the baseline linear attenuation coefficient of the X-ray beam, where water is arbitrarily defined to be zero HU and air defined as −1000 HU.[6] Denser tissue has greater X-ray beam absorption and thus appears bright and has positive values, whereas less dense tissue has less X-ray beam absorption, thus appears dark and has negative values (**Table 1.1**).

Windows

Windowing is the process in which the appearance of a CT image is changed to highlight particular structures. The grayscale component of an image is manipulated via the CT numbers. It is therefore also called gray-level mapping.

Various terminologies that are used in windowing are discussed in subsequent text.

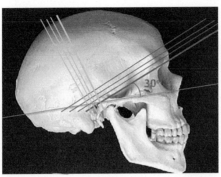

Fig. 1.1 Planes in high-resolution computed tomography temporal bone. Red line: Reid's baseline; Blue lines: axial planes; Green lines: coronal planes.

Table 1.1 Typical Hounsfield units of various tissues

Tissue	Hounsfield units
Air	−1000
Fat	−50 to −100
Water	0
White matter	20–30
Gray matter	37–45
Bone	+1000

Window Width

It is defined as the range of HU that an image contains. A wide window typically has a large number of HU, for example, 400 to 2,000 HU. This would be good for areas where we want to study tissues of various HU together, for example, lungs where we have air, soft tissue, and vessels. Conversely, a narrow window characteristically has a lesser range of HU and is therefore used when areas of interest are of similar attenuation, for example, soft tissues.

Window Level/Window Center

The midpoint of range of HU displayed is referred to as the window level or the window center.

There are mainly the following two types of windows in head and neck.

Soft-Tissue Window

The usual range in soft-tissue window is −125 to +225 HU with window level at +50 HU. It is therefore used for soft tissues such as solid organs.

Bone Window

It is used to study bony details and therefore is very important for studying temporal bone radiology. In the bone window, the window level is +300 HU with a range of −700 to +1300 HU.

Components of a CT Machine

Fig. 1.2 depicts the components of a CT machine.

Filters

Filters in CT machine remove low-energy X-rays, which contribute to image formation but increase the dose of exposure of radiation to the patient, and thus are essential in creating a monochromatic beam.

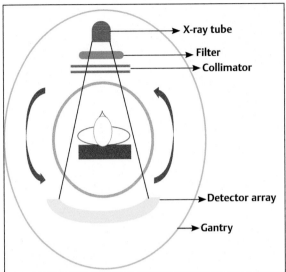

Fig. 1.2 Various components of the CT scan machine.

Collimator

Collimator defines the slice thickness in single-slice scanners and helps to lower radiation dose to the patient.

Detector Array

A single-slice detector has one row of detectors. Multislice detectors have 8 to 128 rows. There are commonly 1,000 to 2,000 detectors in each row.

Gantry

Gantry is a slip-ring which enables continuous rotation of the CT scanner. The rotation time of the gantry is usually between 0.25 and 3 seconds.

Multislice Computed Tomography/Multidetector Computed Tomography

The multislice CT (MSCT), or multidetector CT (MDCT) row, is a CT system with multiple rows of CT detectors to create images in several multiple sections. Advances in MDCT technology with improved software led to significant improvement in the overall quality of cross-sectional images, and two-dimensional (2D) and three-dimensional (3D) reconstructions. MDCT allows us to visualize the anatomic structures of the middle and inner ear in greater detail and accuracy thus aiding in diagnosis and planning prior to surgery. With the advent of MDCT (16 slice onward), it is now possible to obtain multiplanar reconstructions with nearly isotropic resolution.[9] The advantages of MDCT include better dynamic imaging due to faster scanning times, thinner slices, simultaneous acquisition of multiple slices, and it helps in 3D imaging and reconstructions.[10]

High-Resolution Computed Tomography

HRCT uses thin sections of CT images 0.625 to 1 mm slice thickness often with a high spatial frequency reconstruction algorithm. The usual slice thickness in HRCT is 0.6 to 0.7 mm. The resolution of the image means the ability to resolve small objects that are close together on an image as a separate form. The resolution of the image is highly important, as the anatomy of the temporal bone involves minute, small structures in close proximity. HRCT is a scan performed using a high spatial frequency algorithm to accentuate the contrast between tissue of widely differing densities such as air and bone, air and vessels. Collimation is of optimal importance to achieve high resolution. In routine practice, a collimator of 0.6 mm is commonly used during CT of the temporal bone.[9] Collimation wider than 1 mm is not usually used as the resolution is often insufficient. Thicker slices are prone to volume averaging and thus reduce the ability to resolve smaller structures. For 40 to 64 detector scanners, the gantry cycle time is set at 1 cycle or gantry rotation per second. The kilovolt peak (kVp) used in HRCT is usually 120.[11]

Cone-Beam Computed Tomography

Cone-beam CT (CBCT) is a relatively new imaging technique, which was initially developed for angiography and has been used most commonly for dental and maxillofacial evaluation.[12,13] CBCT presents a 3D approach for data acquisition, image display, image reconstruction, and image interpretation. More recently, CBCT has been used for a variety of otologic purposes. The first reported use of CBCT in cochlear implantation was on cadaveric temporal bones by the Freiburg group who demonstrated the superiority of CBCT over the conventional CT in the identification of electrode scalar position.[14]

   CBCT uses a rotating gantry on which an X-ray tube and detector are attached. A cone-shaped X-ray beam is directed through the middle of the temporal bone onto a 2D X-ray detector. In contrast to conventional CT, which uses a narrow fan-shaped beam requiring multiple rotations around the patient to create a volume of data, CBCT requires only a single rotation of a cone-shaped beam (**Fig. 1.3**). In CT scan, HU is proportional to

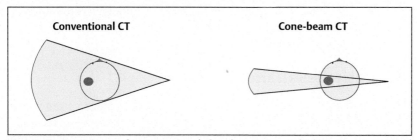

Fig. 1.3 Depiction of conventional fan beam in multidetector computed tomography and cone beam in cone-beam computed tomography preventing radiation exposure to lens.

the degree of X-ray attenuation by the tissue and is assigned to each pixel to show the image that represents the density of the tissue; however, in CBCT, the degree of X-ray attenuation is shown by grayscale (voxel value).[8] The resolution of CBCT is usually between 75 and 300 km which determines the size of the voxels and produces reconstructed images in the three orthogonal planes.[14] The diagnostic importance of CBCT has been proven in the assessment of the position of CIs and visualization of alloplastic middle ear gold, titanium, or platinum implants.

The advantages of CBCT over MSCT/HRCT include higher spatial resolution, reduced metal artifact, shorter acquisition and rapid scanning time, significantly lower radiation dose to the patient, and a reasonable price.[8,15] The most important disadvantage of CBCT is its high sensitivity for motion artifacts as the patient has to hold the head perfectly still during the acquisition time of approximately 40 seconds.[16]

Safety Considerations

The obvious problem with CT is exposure to radiation which is detrimental to various tissues of the body. The biological effects of radiation can be either deterministic or stochastic. The deterministic effects occur only after a threshold dose is exceeded. The stochastic effects may occur at any level of dose.

In the case of HRCT temporal bone, the most detrimental deterministic effect is on the lens as it lies in the same area. Initially, the minimum single dose exposure required to produce a progressive cataract was considered to be 2 Gy.[17] But in the latest statement on tissue reactions issued by the International Commission on Radiological Protection this threshold was decreased to 0.5 Gy.[18] Therefore in HRCT of the temporal bone, the lens should not be in direct X-ray beam. If the lens is in a direct X-ray beam, approximately 0.03 to 0.06 Gy of radiation dose is exposed to the lens when HRCT temporal bone is done. If the patient is positioned such that the lens is not in direct X-ray beam, the dose is approximately 0.003 Gy.[19] It goes without saying that the latter should be tried as far as possible. The stochastic effects include carcinogenesis and mutations, therefore unnecessary radiation exposure should be reduced as much as possible.

CT therefore follows the principle of as low as reasonably achievable (ALARA) with good quality images as needed for diagnosis. Various strategies and protocols are therefore followed by radiologists to minimize the dose of radiation as per the age of the patient, body part being imaged, and the equipment being used.

Magnetic Resonance Imaging

MRI is based on the magnetic resonance property of hydrogen atom which is the most common atom in our body. Hydrogen protons are electrically charged atoms and are considered as magnets with polarity.[20] Each proton spins 360 degrees around its axis with a certain speed and this frequency is called Larmor frequency.

The majority of electromagnets used in the MRI scanner create a magnetic field strength of 1.5 Tesla (T); however, recently manufactured newer machines generate magnetic field strength up to 3 T.[21] For research purposes, magnetic field strength up to 7 T is being used.

1 T = 10,000 gauss and the Earth's magnetic field is approximately 0.5 gauss (i.e., a 3-T machine has a magnetic force 60,000 times that of Earth's magnetic field).

When the patient enters an MRI scanner with a strong magnetic field, hydrogen protons align parallel to the axis of the magnetic field. The MRI scanner also produces radiofrequency pulses exciting the protons to align at an angle to the magnetic field. Milliseconds after removal of the radiofrequency pulse the excited protons in the body relax, and a radiofrequency signal is detected by the receiver in the scanner and is transformed into images.

Relaxation of the protons occurs in following two ways:
1. Realignment of protons with the magnetic field.
2. Dephasing of spinning protons.

Sequences

Based on the type of relaxation, various sequences of MRI are available. On CT images, white means high density in contrast to MRI images where white means bright or high-intensity signal. In MRI generally, the terms low, intermediate, and high signal intensity are frequently used. Depending on the scan protocol, the tissue imaged as dark gray/black is low signal intensity, white is high signal intensity, and gray is intermediate signal intensity (**Fig. 1.4**).

The two basic types of MRI sequences available are: (1) T1-weighted and (2) T2-weighted.

T1-Weighted Sequence

In T1-weighted sequence, the signal is related to the speed of realignment with the magnetic field; the more quickly the protons realign, the greater is the T1 signal. The T1 images predominantly highlight fat tissue within the body and hence fat appears bright on T1 images (**Figs. 1.5** and **1.6**).

T2-Weighted Sequence

In T2-weighted sequence, the signal is related to the speed of proton spin dephasing, that is, the slower the dephasing, the greater is the T2 signal.

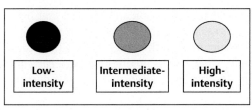

| Low-intensity | Intermediate-intensity | High-intensity |

Fig. 1.4 Color depiction of signals on magnetic resonance imaging. Black: low-intensity signal, gray: intermediate-intensity signal, and white: high-intensity signal.

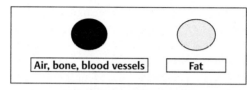

Fig. 1.5 Color depiction of T1-weighted sequence, with black (air, bone, blood vessels) as low-intensity signal and white (fat) as high-intensity signal.

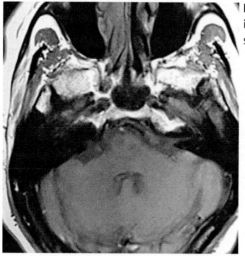

Fig. 1.6 Magnetic resonance imaging brain T1-weighted axial section.

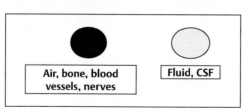

Fig. 1.7 Color depiction Of T2-weighted sequence, with black (air, bone, nerves) as low-intensity signal and white (fluid and cerebrospinal fluid) as high-intensity signal.

The timing of radiofrequency pulse sequences used to make T2 images highlights both fat and water tissue within the body. So water and fat both appear white and bright on T2 images (**Figs. 1.7** and **1.8**). Cerebrospinal fluid (CSF) appears bright and white in T2-weighted images as it is fluid and appears dark in T1 images as it contains no fat.

The other basic sequences available are:

1. Spin echo sequence that aims to remove the effects of the static field but leave the tissue characteristic T2 effect.
2. Gradient echo that is done by using a gradient to rephrase the spins with short TR.

MRI plays a crucial role in the selection of candidates for CIs, and high-resolution sequences using 3D gradient-echo techniques are required to display the fine anatomic structures of the internal auditory canal (IAC), cranial nerves, and the inner ear. 3D techniques that are currently performed at 3.0 T are 3D constructive interference in the steady state

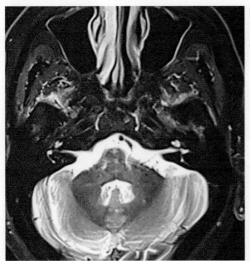

Fig. 1.8 Magnetic resonance imaging brain T2-weighted axial section.

(CISS; Siemens AG, Berlin/Munich, Germany), which is also referred to as fast imaging employing steady-state acquisition with phase cycling (FIESTA-C; General Electric Healthcare, Waukesha, WI).

CISS/FIESTA Sequence

3D CISS/FIESTA is a T2-weighted and an ultrafast pulse sequence that produces high-resolution images that provide higher spatial resolution, clearer and brighter depiction of small structures like cranial nerves, and allows excellent visibility of all the three turns of cochlea, vestibule, and semicircular canal. An image of CSF, endolymph, and perilymph with homogeneous signal intensity is obtained in this technique. This sequence gives an exceptional image contrast between the CSF, perilymph, endolymph fluid to that of nerves, nerve branches, and vessels[22,23] (**Fig. 1.9**).

MRI Planes and Cuts

1.5-T MRI and lately 3-T MRI with 3D reconstruction with eight-channel head coil is commonly used in most centers for MRI. Regularly used sequences in CI imaging are T1 weighted, T2 weighted, and 3D FIESTA/CISS in axial, coronal, and oblique sagittal planes.

Axial and Coronal Plane

Axial T1- and T2-weighted images are obtained through the temporal bone from the arcuate eminence superiorly to the mastoid tip and are perpendicular to the posterior margin of the brainstem described on a midsagittal image.[24] The axial and coronal cuts taken in MRI are of similar angulation as in HRCT temporal bone. Axial CISS or 3D FIESTA images are obtained through the IAC and pons. The usual slice thickness in T1-weighted

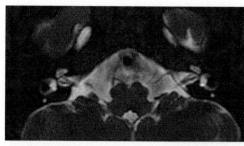

Fig. 1.9 Magnetic resonance imaging temporal bone, axial sections, CISS/FIESTA sequence showing the cochlear and inferior vestibular nerves (in black) contrasting against the cerebrospinal fluid in the internal auditory canal (IAC).

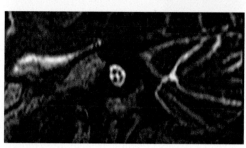

Fig. 1.10 Magnetic resonance imaging temporal bone, CISS/FIESTA sequence oblique sagittal section through internal auditory canal (IAC) showing four nerves.

and T2-weighted sequences is 1 to 3 mm, and that in 3D FIESTA/CISS axial sequence is 1 mm.

Oblique Sagittal Plane

Oblique sagittal images are obtained in the plane perpendicular to the nerves of the IAC, so that we see a cross section of the nerves traversing the IAC (**Fig. 1.10**). These images are typically obtained in CISS/FIESTA sequences, which have been described earlier. This enables us to compare the thickness of the nerves and it will be discussed in detail in the chapters that follow.

Safety Considerations

Due to powerful magnetic and radio-frequency fields, medical device implants with metallic or ferromagnetic components, such as CIs, can create problems during MR scans. Several precautions need to be followed by a cochlear implantee, prior to undergoing an MRI. MRI after CI was initially contraindicated and has been authorized only since 1995 under strict conditions, initially for 0.2-T MRI and then progressively up to 3-T MRI.[25]

MRI examinations performed under different conditions may result in severe injury or device malfunction. The recipient must remove all external components of their CI system before entering a room where an MRI scanner is located. The risks include the potential for device repositioning, localized heating, unusual sounds or sensations, pain or injury, demagnetization, and distortion of the MR image. Another problem posed by MRI post implantation is the artifact generated by either the magnet or the electrode.

Image distortion may spread up to 6 cm around the implant on a 1.5-T MRI and may extend up to 12 cm on a 3-T MRI, when the magnet is left in place.[26] So if we need to image the area near the implanted ear, then it is advisable to remove the magnet so that the artifacts are much lesser. The angle between the MRI magnetic field and the implant's internal magnet must remain less than 90 degree to eliminate the risk of implant magnet demagnetization.[27]

To ensure MRI safety, various CI companies advise removal of the magnet or placing a compression bandage over the implant before the scan. The magnet is easy to remove and replaced if needed. Bandage applied should be 10 cm wide and should pass around the head in at least two layers. Of late, various CI companies have approved for MR scans under specific conditions at 1.5 T and 3 T with the magnet in place developing the feature of MRI compatibility.[28]

Software

The authors in their practice follow the rule of having the soft copy of images that can be studied in detail on any computer available in the hospital. Various softwares are available for this. The authors have personal experience of using Osirix and Horos on iOS systems and RadiAnt on Windows. These softwares allow many controls over the images and are good to plan the surgeries.

References

1. Yigit O, Kalaycik Ertugay C, Yasak AG, Araz Server E. Which imaging modality in cochlear implant candidates? Eur Arch Otorhinolaryngol 2019;276(5):1307–1311
2. Parry DA, Booth T, Roland PS. Advantages of magnetic resonance imaging over computed tomography in preoperative evaluation of pediatric cochlear implant candidates. Otol Neurotol 2005;26(5):976–982
3. Trimble K, Blaser S, James AL, Papsin BC. Computed tomography and/or magnetic resonance imaging before pediatric cochlear implantation? Developing an investigative strategy. Otol Neurotol 2007;28(3):317–324
4. Otake S, Taoka T, Maeda M, Yuh WT. A guide to identification and selection of axial planes in magnetic resonance imaging of the brain. Neuroradiol J 2018;31(4):336–344
5. Honda H, Watanabe K, Kusumoto S, et al. Optimal positioning for CT examinations of the skull base. Experimental and clinical studies. Eur J Radiol 1987;7(4):225–228
6. DenOtter TD, Schubert J. Hounsfield unit. In: StatPearls. Treasure Island, FL: StatPearls Publishing; May 11, 2020
7. Raju TN. The Nobel chronicles. 1979: Allan MacLeod Cormack (b 1924); and Sir Godfrey Newbold Hounsfield (b 1919). Lancet 1999;354(9190):1653
8. Razi T, Niknami M, Alavi Ghazani F. Relationship between Hounsfield unit in CT scan and gray scale in CBCT. J Dent Res Dent Clin Dent Prospect 2014;8(2):107–110
9. Debnath J, George RA, Satija L, et al. High resolution multi detector computed tomography of temporal bone: our experience in a tertiary care service hospital. Indian J Otolaryngol Head Neck Surg 2013;65(Suppl 3):512–519
10. Goldman LW. Principles of CT: multislice CT. J Nucl Med Technol 2008;36(2):57–68, quiz 75–76

11. Swartz JD, Loevner LA, eds. Imaging of the Temporal Bone. 4th ed. Thieme; 2009. Pg 1

12. Demirel O, Kaya E, Üçok CÖ. Evaluation of mastoid pneumatization using cone-beam computed tomography. Oral Radiol 2014;30(1):92–97

13. Sepúlveda I, Schmidt T, Platín E. Use of cone beam computed tomography in the diagnosis of superior semicircular canal dehiscence. J Clin Imaging Sci 2014;4:49

14. Saeed SR, Selvadurai D, Beale T, et al. The use of cone-beam computed tomography to determine cochlear implant electrode position in human temporal bones. Otol Neurotol 2014;35(8): 1338–1344

15. Miracle AC, Mukherji SK. Cone-beam CT of the head and neck, part 1: physical principles. AJNR Am J Neuroradiol 2009;30(6):1088–1095

16. Lemmerling M, De Foer B, eds. Temporal Bone Imaging. Berlin Heidelberg: Springer; 2015

17. Hall EJ, Giaccia AJ. Radiobiology for the Radiologist. 7th ed. Wolters Kluwer Health/Lippincott Williams & Wilkins; 2012

18. Stewart FA, Akleyev AV, Hauer-Jensen M, et al; Authors on behalf of ICRP. ICRP publication 118: ICRP statement on tissue reactions and early and late effects of radiation in normal tissues and organs—threshold doses for tissue reactions in a radiation protection context. Ann ICRP 2012; 41(1-2):1–322

19. Torizuka T, Hayakawa K, Satoh Y, et al. High-resolution CT of the temporal bone: a modified baseline. Radiology 1992;184(1):109–111

20. Berger A. Magnetic resonance imaging. BMJ 2002;324(7328):35

21. Panych LP, Madore B. The physics of MRI safety. J Magn Reson Imaging 2018;47(1):28–43

22. Cavusoglu M, Cılız DS, Duran S, et al. Temporal bone MRI with 3D-FIESTA in the evaluation of facial and audiovestibular dysfunction. Diagn Interv Imaging 2016;97(9):863–869

23. Erdogan N, Altay C, Akay E, et al. MRI assessment of internal acoustic canal variations using 3D-FIESTA sequences. Eur Arch Otorhinolaryngol 2013;270(2):469–475

24. Kopřiva J, Žižka J. Temporal Bone CT and MRI Anatomy. Springer International Publishing; 2015. Pg 157

25. Deneuve S, Loundon N, Leboulanger N, Rouillon I, Garabedian EN. Cochlear implant magnet displacement during magnetic resonance imaging. Otol Neurotol 2008;29(6):789–190

26. Orús Dotú C, Venegas Pizarro MdelP, De Juan Beltrán J, De Juan Delago M. Reimplantación coclear en el mismo oído: hallazgos, peculiaridades de la técnica quirúrgica y complicaciones. [Cochlear reimplantation in the same ear: Findings, peculiarities of the surgical technique and complications] Acta Otorrinolaringol Esp 2010;61(2):106–117

27. Bawazeer N, Vuong H, Riehm S, Veillon F, Charpiot A. Magnetic resonance imaging after cochlear implants. J Otol 2019;14(1):22–25

28. Precautions to Take for Children with Cochlear Implants. ENT for Children. Published December 20, 2017. Accessed May 31, 2020. https://entforchildren.com/precautions-take-children-cochlear-implants/

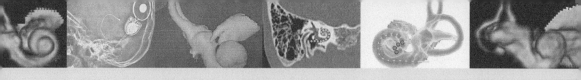

Chapter 2

Radiology of External and Middle Ear Pertaining to Cochlear Implant

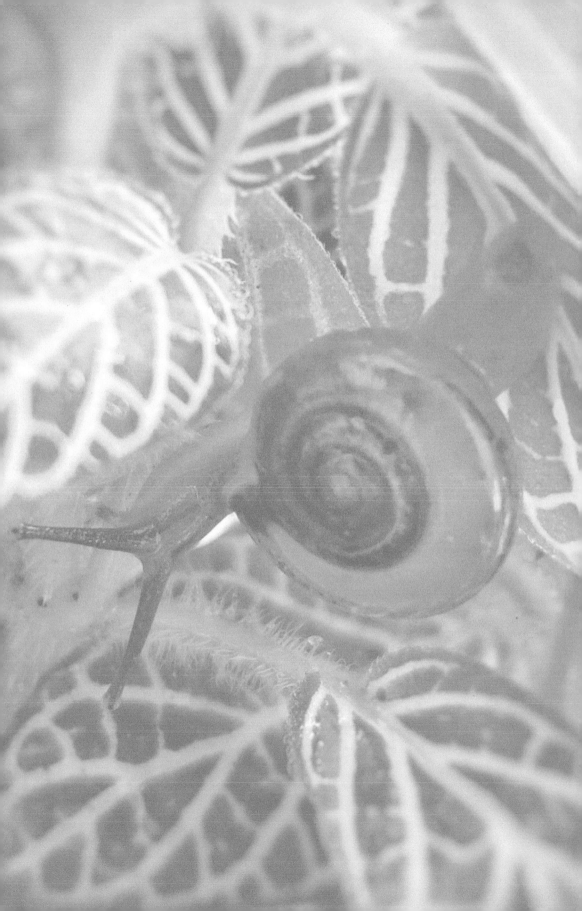

2 Radiology of External and Middle Ear Pertaining to Cochlear Implant

Introduction

Though cochlear implantation is a surgery that involves the inner ear, the route for entry in the inner ear is through the middle ear. Malformations of the external ear also impact this path which leads to the cochlea. In fact, radiology is very important when we want to predict many things related to this surgery as we go through the various parts of the middle ear cleft.

In this chapter, author will be discussing in detail about various aspects of radiology of the external and middle ear which plays an important role in cochlear implant surgery. For this purpose, author will be discussing various sections of high-resolution computed tomography (HRCT) temporal bone in relation to the above. By convention, the axial sections have to be read from superior to inferior and coronal sections from anterior to posterior.

Axial Sections

When we start reading the axial sections from superior to inferior, the first part of the middle ear cleft which we see is the mastoid air cells (**Figs. 2.1** and **2.2**). This pneumatization may vary from sclerotic to diploic to well-pneumatized to hyperpneumatized (**Fig. 2.22**). Operation on a sclerotic mastoid with a small antrum may sometimes be more time-consuming. At the same time, a hyperpneumatized mastoid may have a dehiscent facial nerve opening in a cell (**Fig. 2.22**).

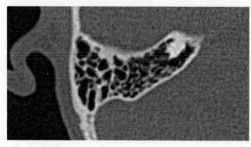

Fig. 2.1 HRCT temporal bone, axial section, bone window. Superior most cut showing only mastoid air cells.

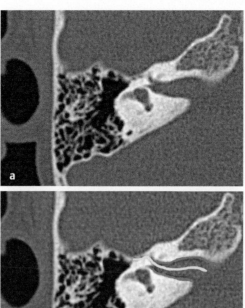

Fig. 2.2 (a, b) HRCT temporal bone, axial section, bone window, at the level of internal acoustic canal (IAC) shows mastoid air cells, with corresponding colored structures, (█ dark green) internal acoustic meatus and (█ yellow) facial nerve–meatal and labyrinthine segment.

The first section where we start seeing the ossicles is usually at the level where we see the "signet ring" appearance of the lateral semicircular canal (LSCC) (**Fig. 2.3**). The head of malleus is the anterior bony shadow and the body of incus is the posterior bony shadow. They both, as we know, occupy the attic (epitympanum).

As we go inferiorly, with every cut we start seeing various appearances of ossicles including the well-known "ice cream cone appearance." Also, the same cuts show the tympanic segment of the facial nerve (**Fig. 2.4**). The facial nerve will be discussed in detail later.

Going inferiorly, we see tensor tympani anteriorly, hooking up from processus cochleariformis going toward the neck of the malleus. In the same section, we can see stapes suprastructure, sinus tympani, and vertical segment of the facial nerve (**Fig. 2.5**).

In the next section (as depicted in **Fig. 2.6**), we can identify the beginning of the external auditory canal (EAC), chorda tympani, and vertical segment of facial nerve. We can also use this section to calculate the facial recess approach. Stapedius can also be seen arising from the pyramid and going toward the stapes neck. Impression of the round window is seen as a hypodense area next to the basal turn of the cochlea.

Fig. 2.7 shows internal carotid artery and eustachian tube anteriorly and subcochlear canaliculus posteriorly. This relation is important because surgeons have put electrodes in each of these three places. The subcochlear canaliculus has been divided into three types depending on pneumatization.

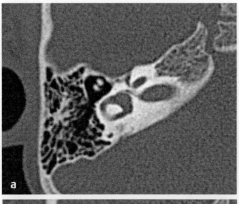

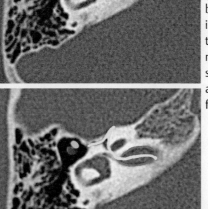

Fig. 2.3 **(a, b)** HRCT temporal bone, axial section, bone window at the level of signet ring appearance shows the start of ossicles, with corresponding colored structures, (█ light green) head of malleus, (█ pink) body of incus, (█ dark green) internal acoustic meatus with the facial nerve, (█ yellow) meatal segment, labyrinthine segment, geniculate ganglion, and tympanic segment of the facial nerve.

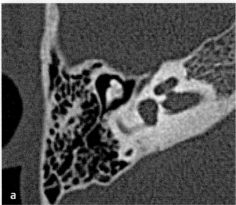

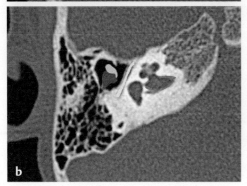

Fig. 2.4 **(a, b)** HRCT temporal bone, axial section, bone window shows ice cream cone appearance of ossicles, with corresponding colored structures, (█ light green) head of malleus, (█ pink) body of incus with short process pointing to the facial nerve, (█ yellow) tympanic segment of the facial nerve, and (█ dark green) internal acoustic meatus.

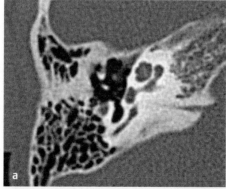

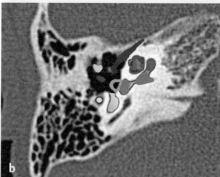

Fig. 2.5 (a, b) HRCT temporal bone, axial section, bone window at the level of cochlea with all the three turns, with corresponding colored structures showing, (light green) neck of the malleus, (pink) long process of incus, (light blue) stapes, (yellow) mastoid segment of facial nerve, (purple) cochlea, (light brown) saccule, (light orange) sinus tympani, (dark brown) tensor tympani, and (dark green) fundus of the internal acoustic meatus.

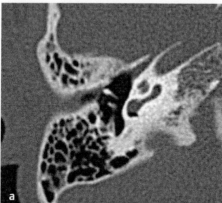

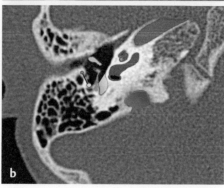

Fig. 2.6 (a, b) HRCT temporal bone, axial section, bone window shows (light green) handle of malleus, (pink) long process and lenticular process of incus, (light blue) head and neck of stapes, (purple) apical, middle, and basal turn of the cochlea with round window, (yellow) mastoid segment of the facial nerve, (light pink) chorda tympani, facial recess indicated by ■ black line, and sinus tympani by light orange each on either side of the pyramid, (orange) stapedius tendon (from pyramid to stapes), (dark blue) jugular bulb, and (red) internal carotid artery.

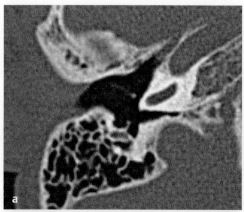

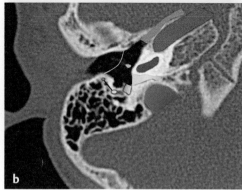

Fig. 2.7 (a, b) HRCT temporal bone, axial section, bone window, with corresponding colored structures shows (light green) handle of malleus, (yellow) mastoid segment of the facial nerve, (light pink) chorda tympani, facial recess indicated by black line and sinus tympani by light orange each on either side of the pyramid, (purple) basal turn of cochlea, (light yellow) subcochlear canaliculus, (light violet) tympanic membrane, (light brown) eustachian tube, (dark blue) jugular bulb, and (red) internal carotid artery.

Marchioni et al[1] divided subcochlear canaliculus into the following three types:

- Type A: Deep pneumatization with communication between the middle ear and petrous apex.
- Type B: Limited pneumatization going below the cochlea.
- Type C: No pneumatization below the cochlea.

Type A is the most risky where surgeons may confuse it with cochlear lumen. Also, many times internal carotid artery may be dehiscent in the type A subcochlear canaliculus.

Another structure that might be prominent at this level is the jugular bulb. If it is too high, it may prove to be a hindrance while doing a posterior tympanotomy or visualizing the round window or doing cochleostomy. Therefore, this needs to be identified well.

One section inferior (**Fig. 2.8**), we see the well-defined bulge of promontory and anterior to it the bulge of internal carotid artery. Anterior to the carotid is the eustachian tube. Incidentally, sometimes EAC may show wax (as shown in **Fig. 2.8**). Rest of the structures are similar.

As we go inferiorly (**Fig. 2.9**), the bulge of carotid becomes more prominent and so do the hypotympanic cells depending on the pneumatization. Jugular bulb may be variably seen depending on its prominence.

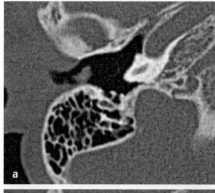

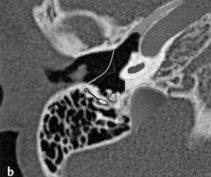

Fig. 2.8 (a, b) HRCT temporal bone, axial section, bone window, with corresponding colored structures shows, (■ purple) basal turn of the cochlea, (yellow) mastoid segment of the facial nerve, (■ light pink) chorda tympani, facial recess indicated by ■ black line and sinus tympani by ▮ light orange each on either side of the pyramid, (light yellow) subcochlear canaliculus, (■ light violet) tympanic membrane, (■ light brown) eustachian tube, (■ dark blue) jugular bulb, and (■ red) internal carotid artery.

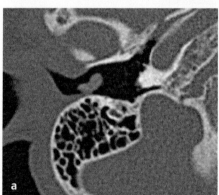

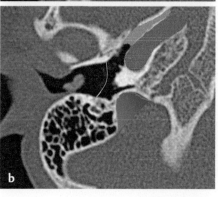

Fig. 2.9 (a, b) HRCT temporal bone, axial section, bone window, with corresponding colored structures shows, (■ light violet) tympanic membrane, (■ light brown) eustachian tube, (■ dark blue) jugular bulb, and (■ red) internal carotid artery.

Coronal Sections

By convention, coronal sections are read from anterior to posterior. The anterior most section will usually show only internal carotid artery inferiorly with its bulge in the middle ear and tensor tympani superiorly (**Fig. 2.10**). As we go just posterior, we usually start seeing cochlea and segments of the facial nerve as well (**Figs. 2.11, 2.12, 2.13, and 2.14**). More posterior sections (**Figs. 2.14** and **2.15**) show the scutum, malleus, and EAC and variable pneumatization of mastoid air cells. Going posteriorly (**Figs. 2.13, 2.14, 2.15, and 2.16**) we see the various ossicles with oval window. Usually just one section posterior (**Fig. 2.17**) to one with the oval window we start seeing the round window. The posterior most cuts when almost everything important in the middle and inner ear has finished shows the vertical segment of the facial nerve (**Figs. 2.18, 2.19, and 2.20**).

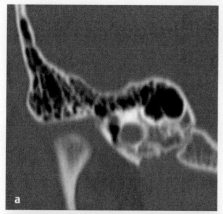
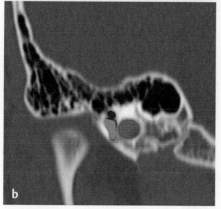

Fig. 2.10 (a, b) HRCT temporal bone, coronal section, bone window, anterior most cut shows temporo-mandibular joint, with corresponding colored structures, (■ dark brown) tensor tympani muscle, (■ light brown) eustachian tube, and (■ red) internal carotid artery.

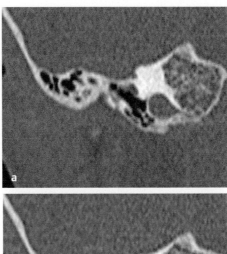

Fig. 2.11 (a, b) HRCT temporal bone, coronal section, bone window, with corresponding colored structures shows, (yellow) geniculate ganglion of the facial nerve, (dark brown) tensor tympani muscle, and (red) internal carotid artery.

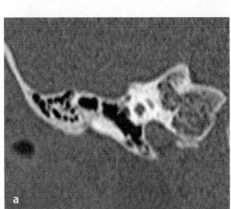

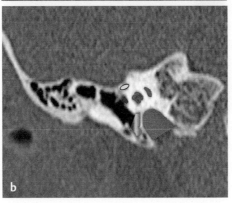

Fig. 2.12 (a, b) HRCT temporal bone, coronal section, bone window, with corresponding colored structures shows, (purple) cochlea, (yellow) facial nerve, (dark brown) tensor tympani muscle, (shaded green) hypotympanic air cells, and (red) internal carotid artery.

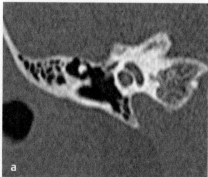

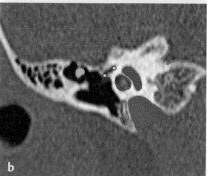

Fig. 2.13 (a, b) HRCT temporal bone, coronal section, bone window, with corresponding colored structures shows, (light green) head of malleus, (purple) cochlea, (dark green) internal acoustic meatus, (yellow) tympanic and labyrinthine segment of the facial nerve (snake eye appearance), (dark brown) tensor tympani muscle, (shaded green) hypotympanic air cells, and (red) internal carotid artery.

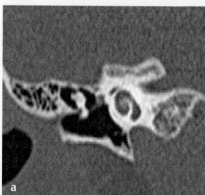

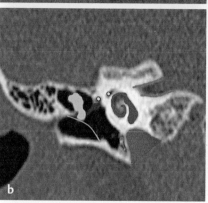

Fig. 2.14 (a, b) HRCT temporal bone, coronal section, bone window, with corresponding colored structures shows, (light green) head, neck of malleus in anterior epitympanum, (purple) cochlea, (dark green) internal acoustic meatus, (yellow) tympanic and labyrinthine segment of the facial nerve (snake eye appearance), (light violet) tympanic membrane, (dark brown) tensor tympani, (shaded green) hypotympanic air cells, and (red) internal carotid artery.

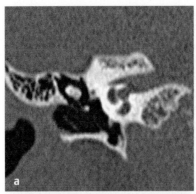

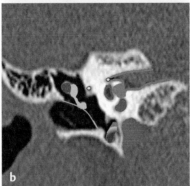

Fig. 2.15 (a, b) HRCT temporal bone, coronal section, bone window, with corresponding colored structures shows, (■ light green) malleus, (■ pink) incus, (■ purple) cochlea, (■ dark green) internal acoustic meatus, (■ yellow) tympanic and labyrinthine segment of the facial nerve, (■ light violet) tympanic membrane, (■ shaded green) hypotympanic air cells, and (■ red) internal carotid artery.

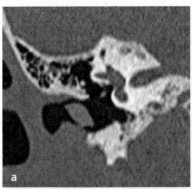

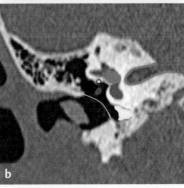

Fig. 2.16 (a, b) HRCT temporal bone, coronal section, bone window, with corresponding colored structures shows, (■ pink) long process of incus, (■ light blue) stapes footplate, (■ purple) basal turn of cochlea, (■ dark green) internal acoustic meatus, (■ yellow) tympanic segment of the facial nerve (pear under tree appearance), (■ light brown) saccule, (■ light violet) tympanic membrane, and (■ light yellow) subcochlear canaliculus.

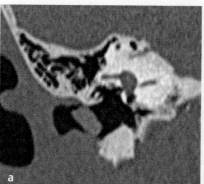

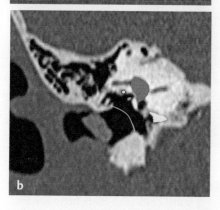

Fig. 2.17 (a, b) HRCT temporal bone, coronal section, bone window, with corresponding colored structures shows, (▮ light blue) stapes, (▮ yellow) tympanic segment of the facial nerve, (▮ light brown) vestibule, (▮ light yellow) subcochlear canaliculus, and (▮ light violet) tympanic membrane.

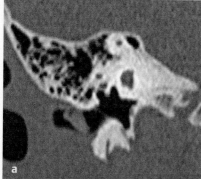

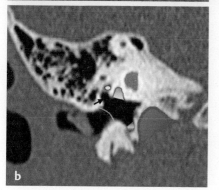

Fig. 2.18 (a, b) HRCT temporal bone, coronal section, bone window, with corresponding colored structures shows, (▮ yellow) tympanic segment of the facial nerve, and sinus tympani by ▮ light orange each on either side of the pyramid, (▮ shaded green) hypotympanic air cells, (▮ light violet) tympanic membrane, (▮ light brown) vestibule, and (▮ dark blue) jugular bulb.

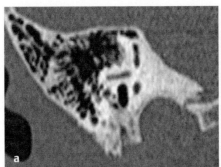

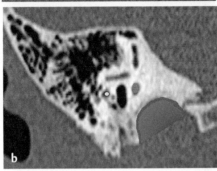

Fig. 2.19 (a, b) HRCT temporal bone, coronal section, bone window, with corresponding colored structures shows, (yellow) mastoid segment of the facial nerve, (light brown) vestibule, and (dark blue) jugular bulb.

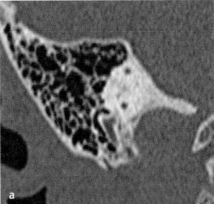

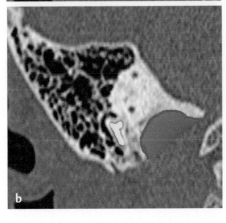

Fig. 2.20 (a, b) HRCT temporal bone, coronal section, bone window, with corresponding colored structures shows, (yellow) mastoid segment of the facial nerve and (dark blue) jugular bulb.

Oblique Sagittal Reconstruction

Fig. 2.21 shows an oblique sagittal image. It is not a true section but can be reconstructed. The authors in their experience find this cut to be really useful because it shows lots of structures and their relations in one section. It shows various parts of the facial nerve: the labyrinthine segment, major part of the tympanic segment, second genu, and the whole vertical segment. It also shows the oval window and round window, jugular and carotid artery and these relations are therefore a good guide for surgery. Various parts of the inner ear are also visible in this section which will be discussed in the relevant chapter.

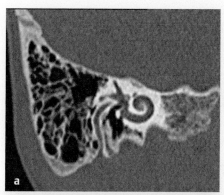

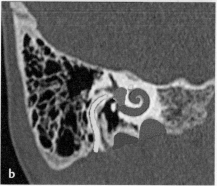

Fig. 2.21 (a, b) HRCT temporal bone, oblique sagittal reconstruction shows (yellow) labyrinthine, tympanic, second genu, and mastoid segment of the facial nerve; (■ purple) cochlea; (■ red) internal carotid artery; (■ dark blue) jugular bulb; (■ light blue) stapes at oval window; (■ light brown) saccule; and white arrow pointing to round window.

Special Variants to Be Considered

Mastoid Pneumatization

The pneumatization can vary from sclerosed to extensive pneumatization. Both the extremes require the surgeon to be more careful. In a sclerosed mastoid, the surgeon may have issues finding the antrum or antrum may sometimes be too small (**Fig. 2.22a**). In an extensively pneumatized mastoid (**Fig. 2.22b**), sometimes the facial nerve may be dehiscent in one of the cells and if that cell is opened, the facial nerve may get exposed (**Fig. 2.23**).

Sinus Plate

Forward lying sigmoid sinus can lead to issues with cortical mastoidectomy and posterior tympanotomy, and the surgeon should look out for this to be prepared for this kind of scenario (**Fig. 2.22a**: same as used for sclerosed mastoid in previous section). If the surgeon misses to recognize this variant preoperatively, there is a high chance of inadvertently injuring the sigmoid sinus. Many times this is associated with a high jugular bulb which, if present, may create additional problems.

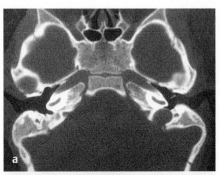
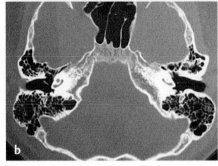

Fig. 2.22 HRCT temporal bone, axial section shows **(a)** sclerosed mastoid and **(b)** hyperpneumatized mastoid.

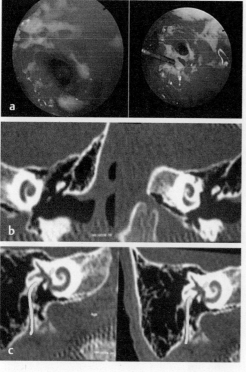

Fig. 2.23 HRCT temporal bone shows dehiscent facial nerve **(a)** intraoperatively during posterior tympanotomy. **(b** and **c)** HRCT temporal bone, oblique sagittal reconstructed image showing dehiscent mastoid segment of the facial nerve (yellow) in a hyperpneumatized mastoid air cell.

Tegmen (Low-Lying Dura)

Level of the dural plate is important in all mastoid surgeries. By definition, if the level of tegmen is lower than the level of the superior semicircular canal, then it is considered to be low-lying dural plate (**Fig. 2.24**).

Korner's Septum

Korner's septum is the persistent petrosquamous suture. It is many times mistaken as the medial wall of mastoid antrum. This can lead to complications such as facial nerve injury. This is specially a possibility in cochlear implant surgery as the surgeon is not visualizing the middle ear. To avoid this, it is important to identify it preoperatively with the help of radiology (**Fig. 2.25**). Intraoperatively, the surgeon should keep in mind the depth of supposed antrum and identification of lateral semicircular canal to confirm that he or she has entered mastoid antrum.

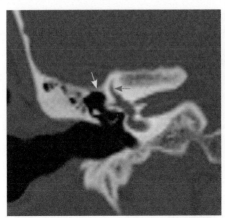

Fig. 2.24 HRCT temporal bone coronal section shows (yellow arrow) low-lying tegmen plate and (red arrow) superior semicircular canal.

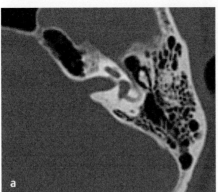

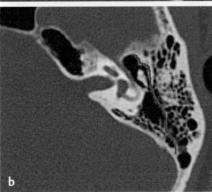

Fig. 2.25 (a, b) HRCT temporal bone, axial section shows (in pink) Korner's septum.

Facial Nerve

Facial nerve may be dehiscent, anomalous, or duplicated. It is known to be dehiscent in the tympanic segment in approximately one-third of patients.[2] As we saw in the section on mastoid pneumatization, the vertical segment may be dehiscent in one of the nerves (**Fig. 2.23**). It is known to be anomalous especially in association with certain malformations such as cochlear hypoplasias. This will be discussed in detail in the chapter on malformations. Facial nerve is also known to be duplicated (**Fig. 2.26**) and if this happens in the vertical segment, it may lead to narrowing of facial recess and also lead to injury during posterior tympanotomy if the surgeon is not careful.

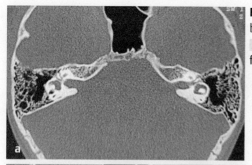
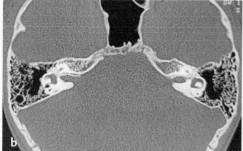

Fig. 2.26   (a, b) HRCT temporal bone, axial sections shows (in yellow) bilateral duplicated facial nerve.

Facial Recess

Standard transmastoid posterior tympanotomy (Facial Recess or Wullstein's Window) is the classical approach followed in cochlear implantation surgery. Facial recess is a triangular space of mastoid air cells delineated by the mastoid segment of the facial nerve medially, chorda tympani nerve anterolaterally, and fossa incudis superiorly. The width of the facial recess is measured by perpendicularly drawing a line from the anterolateral part of the facial nerve to the chorda tympani on axial sections of HRCT temporal bone, at the level of the round window, as shown in the **Figs. 2.6 (a, b)** and **2.27 (a, b)**. If the distance between the facial nerve and chorda tympani is less than 1 mm, it is considered as a narrow facial recess.[3] As both access to the cochlea and the risk of facial nerve damage depend on the width of the facial recess, preoperative assessment of facial recess radiologically becomes a necessity.

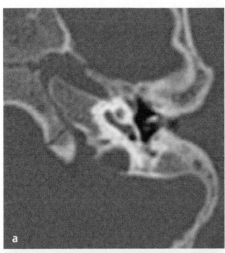

Fig. 2.27 (a, b) HRCT temporal bone axial section, shows narrow facial recess (black line) less than 1 mm measured between facial nerve (yellow) and chorda tympani (■ pink).

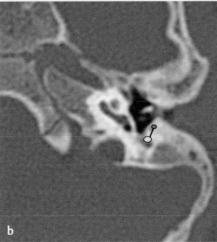

Aberrant/Anomalous Carotid Artery

Aberrant internal carotid artery is a rare anomaly seen more commonly on the right side and mostly in females. It is an enlarged inferior tympanic branch of the ascending pharyngeal artery commonly seen when there is agenesis or underdevelopment of the vertical portion of the carotid canal.[4] This aberrant vessel enters the hypotympanum via an enlarged inferior tympanic canaliculus and courses along the medial aspect of the middle ear, passing across the promontory (basal turn of the cochlea) (**Fig. 2.28**)[5] to join the horizontal part of the carotid canal. Identification of this anomaly on radiology preoperatively is important, as injury to this vessel during cochleostomy could be life-threatening.

Jugular Bulb

Jugular bulb on one side may be more prominent than the jugular bulb on the other. Usually, the right-side jugular bulb is more prominent. Many criteria have been used to define a high jugular bulb, viz above the level of the posterior semicircular canal (**Fig. 2.29**), above the level of the basal turn of the cochlea, or above the level of inferior tympanic annulus. A jugular bulb extending up to the basal turn of the cochlea may obliterate the round window niche (**Fig. 2.30**) and thus reduce visualization and accessibility to round window during cochlear implantation.

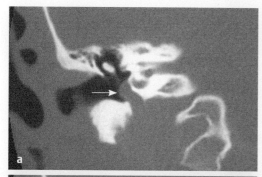

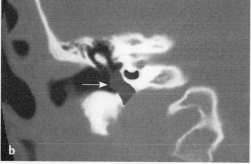

Fig. 2.28 (a, b) HRCT temporal bone, coronal section shows (in ■ red)—Aberrant internal carotid artery coursing over (in ■ purple)—basal turn of the cochlea. White arrow points towards the bulging of aberrant internal carotid artery into middle ear.

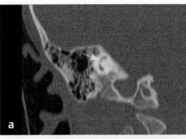

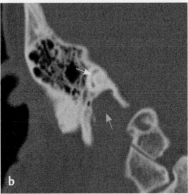

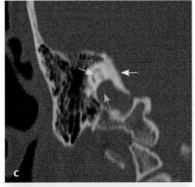

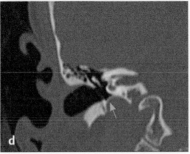

Fig. 2.29 HRCT temporal bone, coronal section shows (in ■ blue) types of jugular bulb (blue arrow) in relation to posterior semicircular canal (yellow arrow) and in ▨ green internal acoustic meatus (white arrow). **(a)** Type 1, **(b)** Type 2, **(c)** Type 3, **(d)** jugular bulb without dehiscence into the middle ear. *(Continued)*

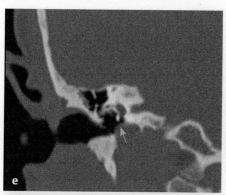

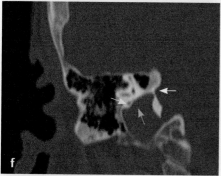

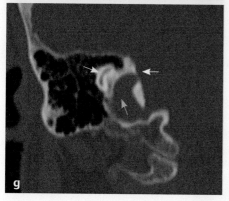

Fig. 2.29 *(Continued)* HRCT temporal bone, coronal section shows (in ■ blue) types of jugular bulb in relation to posterior semicircular canal (yellow arrow) and (in ■ green) internal acoustic meatus (white arrow). **(e)** jugular bulb dehiscence into the middle ear, **(f, g)** type 4a, and **(h)** type 4b. *(Continued)*

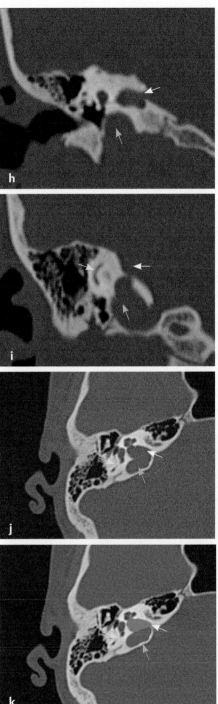

Fig. 2.29 *(Continued)* HRCT temporal bone, coronal section shows (in ▓ blue) types of jugular bulb in relation to posterior semicircular canal (yellow arrow) and (in ▓ green) internal acoustic meatus (white arrow). **(h, i, j, k)** type 4b.

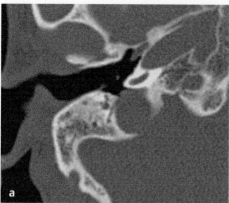

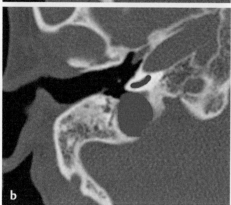

Fig. 2.30 (a, b) HRCT temporal bone, axial section shows high jugular bulb (in ■ blue) above the level of the basal turn of cochlea (in ■ purple).

Manjila and Semaan outlined a detailed classification for position of jugular bulb in relation to the posterior semicircular canal and internal acoustic meatus[6] (**Fig. 2.29**), on coronal sections of CT imaging and divided into 5 types. According to this classification Type 1 is no jugular bulb (**Fig. 2.29a**). Type 2 is jugular bulb positioned below the inferior margin of the posterior SCC (**Fig. 2.29b**) which is further divided into Type 2A (Without dehiscence into the middle ear (**Fig. 2.29b** and **d**) and Type 2B (With dehiscence into the middle ear (**Fig. 2.29b** and **e**). Type 3 is jugular bulb extending between inferior margin of posterior SCC and inferior margin of IAC (**Fig. 2.29c**). Type 3 is further divided into Type 3 A (Without dehiscence into the middle ear (**Fig. 2.29c** and **d**)) and Type 3 B (With dehiscence into the middle ear (**Fig. 2.29c** and **c**)). Type 4 is when jugular bulb extends above the inferior margin of IAC, if there is no dehiscence into the IAC (**Fig. 2.29 f**and **g**) it is considered as Type 4 A and Type 4B if there is dehiscence into the IAC (**Fig. 2.29h, i, j, k**). If there is a combination of dehiscence it is considered Type 5.

External Auditory Canal Atresia

EAC atresia and microtia change a lot of things in cochlear implants, right from evaluation to surgery and then fitting the external processor. Facial nerve is commonly anomalous and ossicles dysplastic (**Fig. 2.31a**). These two things specially make a lot of difference to surgery. A smaller middle ear may also make things difficult (**Fig. 2.31b**). Many surgeons would like to use navigation system in such cases to avoid complications.

Emissary Vein

The mastoid emissary vein, petrosquamosal sinus, occipital emissary vein, and posterior condylar vein are the major posterior fossa emissary veins which contribute in extracranial venous drainage of the posterior fossa dural sinuses. The mastoid emissary vein runs between the sigmoid sinus and posterior auricular vein or occipital vein by crossing the mastoid foramen (**Fig. 2.32a–d**). The petrosquamosal sinus arises from the transverse sinus just before its junction with the sigmoid sinus and drains into the retromandibular vein. Most of the emissary veins are usually small, asymptomatic and disappear with time; however, some persist and increase in size in patients with high-flow vascular malformations.[7] Petrosquamosal sinus are rare in humans and are usually associated with

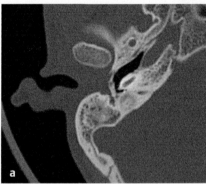
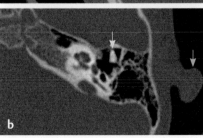

Fig. 2.31 HRCT temporal bone axial section, shows **(a)** Right Microtia with EAC atresia, **(b)** Left microtia (blue arrow) with EAC atresia and Dysplastic ossicles (yellow arrow).

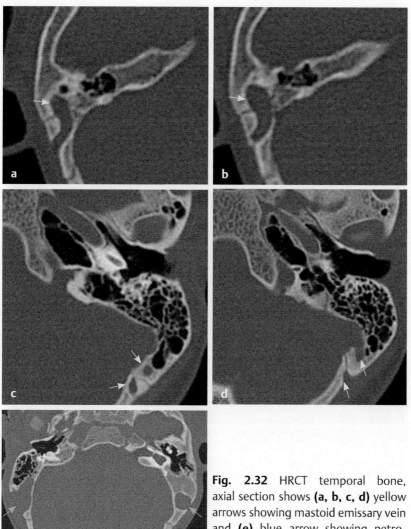

Fig. 2.32 HRCT temporal bone, axial section shows **(a, b, c, d)** yellow arrows showing mastoid emissary vein and **(e)** blue arrow showing petro-squamous sinus.

craniofacial syndromes with craniosynostosis, semicircular canal dysplasia such as charge syndrome (**Fig. 2.32e**).[7] Emissary veins are considered large if diameter is more than 3.5 mm. These emissary veins need to be identified via imaging prior to mastoid or cochlear implant surgery as its sacrifice could cause life-threatening bleed during surgery and adequate precautions need to be taken to control the bleed. Previous studies in the literature have reported excessive use of surgical materials such as bone wax to control hemostasis that can migrate,[8] and can predispose to complications such as venous thrombosis.

Skull Thickness

Proper placement of the receiver stimulator package of the implant requires drilling well with adequate depth depending on the model and the company of the implant. Therefore, getting an idea of skull thickness at the proposed site of well is good to avoid dural exposure if possible. This helps in getting adequate depth for the implant as well as avoiding unnecessary exposure of dura. **Fig. 2.33** shows comparison between a skull with normal thickness and another with areas of thin skull that, if possible, should be avoided for the well.

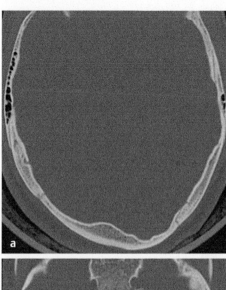

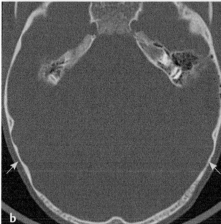

Fig. 2.33 HRCT temporal bone, axial section shows **(a)** normal skull thickness, **(b)** thin skull (yellow arrows).

References

1. Marchioni D, Alicandri-Ciufelli M, Pothier DD, Rubini A, Presutti L. The round window region and contiguous areas: endoscopic anatomy and surgical implications. Eur Arch Otorhinolaryngol 2015;272(5):1103–1112

2. Bulja D, Stojanov D, Ignjatovic J, Bjelakovic M, Popovic J, Ignjatovic N. The incidence of dehiscence of the tympanic segment of the facial nerve canal estimated with computed tomography. In RAD Conference Proceedings. 2016 Jun 15

3. Wang L, Yang J, Jiang C, Zhang D. Cochlear implantation surgery in patients with narrow facial recess. Acta Otolaryngol 2013;133(9): 935–938

4. Offiah CE, Ramsden RT, Gillespie JE. Imaging appearances of unusual conditions of the middle and inner ear. Br J Radiol 2008;81(966):504–514

5. Alharethy S. Aberrant internal carotid artery in the middle ear. Ann Saudi Med 2013;33(2): 194–196

6. Manjila S, Bazil T, Kay M, Udayasankar UK, Semaan M. Jugular bulb and skull base pathologies: proposal for a novel classification system for jugular bulb positions and microsurgical implications. Neurosurg Focus 2018;45(1):E5

7. Pekçevik Y, Pekçevik R. Why should we report posterior fossa emissary veins? Diagn Interv Radiol 2014;20(1):78–81

8. Hadeishi H, Yasui N, Suzuki A. Mastoid canal and migrated bone wax in the sigmoid sinus: technical report. Neurosurgery 1995;36(6):1220–1223, discussion 1223–1224

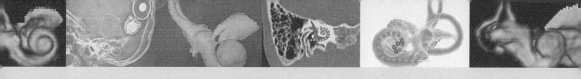

Chapter 3

Radiology of Normal Inner Ear and Internal Acoustic Canal

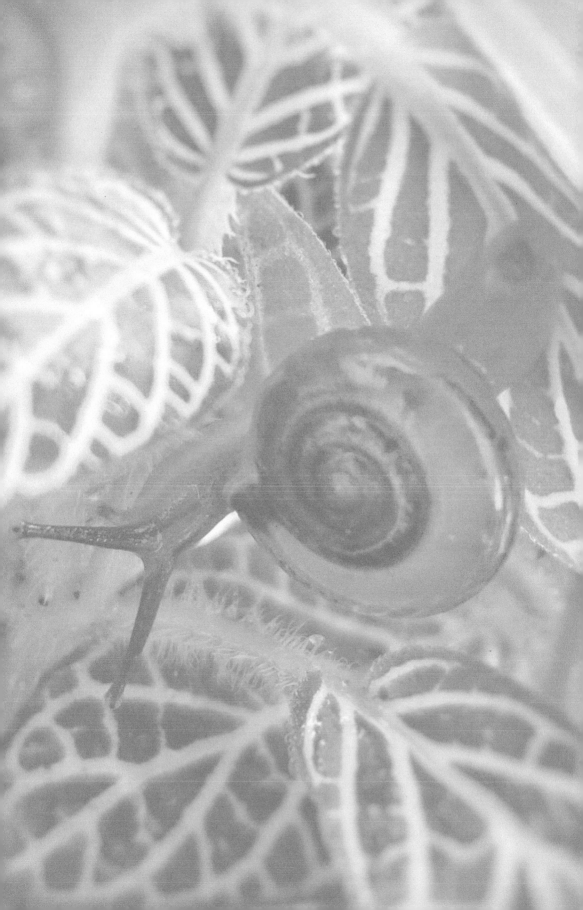

3 Radiology of Normal Inner Ear and Internal Acoustic Canal

Introduction

To understand the inner ear radiology, it is important to understand the normal anatomy. The inner ear is divided into cochlear and vestibular parts. The cochlea is anterior to the internal acoustic canal (IAC) while the vestibular part is posterior to the canal. The vestibular part consists of the utricle, the saccule, the three semicircular canals (SCCs), and the endolymphatic sac and duct. The cochlear part has the cochlea and the cochlear aqueduct.

It is important to understand the anatomy of the cochlea with respect to radiology (**Fig. 3.1**). The cochlea is a snail-shaped spiral structure consisting of 2.5 to 2.75 turns: basal, middle, and apical turns. The cochlea coils around an axis called the modiolus. Modiolus is a bony structure and therefore can be visualized on high-resolution computed tomography (HRCT) temporal bone. It can also be visualized in CISS/FIESTA magnetic resonance imaging (MRI) in contrast to the bright signal of fluid in the cochlea. Some authors have described that the modiolus looks like a "crown." This may get distorted in malformed cochlea. Various septations arise from the modiolus and go to the outer wall, such that they divide the cochlea into the basal, middle, and apical turns. CISS/FIESTA MRI also shows the bright signal of scala tympani and vestibuli, divided by the osseous spiral lamina (OSL). A well done HRCT will also be able to show the division between scala tympani and scala vestibuli. The cochlear nerve endings in a normal

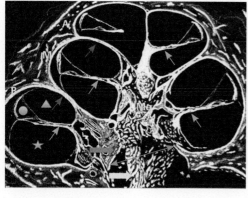

Fig. 3.1 Schematic diagram of histopathological section of the cochlea, B: basal turn of cochlea, M: middle turn of the cochlea, A: apical turn of the cochlea, Mo: modiolus, blue star - scala tympani, blue triangle - scala vestibuli, blue circle - scala media, red arrow - interscalar septations, blue arrow - osseous spiral lamina, pink arrow - lamina cribrosa, green arrow - cochlear aperture, yellow arrow - cochlear nerve.

cochlea are placed in the modiolus. They leave the cochlea to enter the IAC through the cochlear aperture. The cochlear aperture is a small opening through which the cochlea is connected to the IAC. Cochlear aperture is also called a bony cochlear nerve canal (BCNC). Histopathologically, there is a thin plate of bone dividing the cochlea and IAC which is pierced by cochlear nerve fibers in a sieve-like manner. This bony partition is called lamina cribrosa. It can be visualized in a good-quality HRCT temporal bone sections and authors experience the absence of lamina cribrosa is a major factor to predict cerebrospinal fluid (CSF) gusher during surgery. The other two important factors which predict perilymph ooze or CSF gusher are aqueducts of cochlea and vestibule.

Here are a few of the important structures along with their dimensions to describe a normal inner ear:

1. Cochlea having a minimum of 2.5 turns.
2. Cochlear duct length more than 25 mm.
3. If a vestibular aqueduct is more than 1.5 mm at its midpoint, it is considered as an enlarged vestibular aqueduct (Valvassori criteria).[1]
4. Endolymphatic duct is considered to be enlarged when its diameter exceeds double that of the adjacent portion of the posterior semicircular canal (SCC) (Wilson criteria).[2]
5. BCNC: if it is less than 1.4 mm, it is suggestive of cochlear nerve hypoplasia or aplasia. If it is more than 3 mm, it is suggestive of higher chances of CSF gusher/absent modiolus.[3]

For the rest of the temporal bone, MRI has limited indications (such as tumors or complications of otitis media); however, it is imperative to get an MRI of the brain and temporal bone for evaluating patients who are being planned for cochlear implants. Brain needs to be evaluated to rule out any central pathology like acoustic neuromas or calcifications/cystic demyelination post cytomegalovirus (CMV) infection.

In the following text, authors will be discussing various sections pertaining to inner ear radiology.

Axial Sections

As discussed previously, axial sections are the most important in the radiology of temporal bones. By convention, they are read from superior to inferior.

The first part of the inner ear to appear is the dome of the superior SCC (**Fig. 3.2**). As we go inferior, the anterior (ampullated) and posterior (non-ampullated) limbs of superior SCC are visualized (**Fig. 3.3**). More inferior, we are able to see the posterior SCC joining the superior SCC at crus commune (**Fig. 3.4**). Just as the posterior SCC is seen to be separate from the crus commune we are usually able to see the starting of the IAC. CISS/FIESTA MRI at the same level might show two nerves in IAC, viz facial nerve (anteriorly) and superior vestibular nerve (posteriorly) (**Fig. 3.5**).

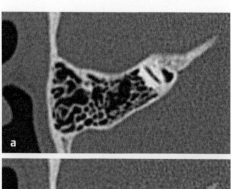

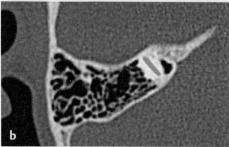

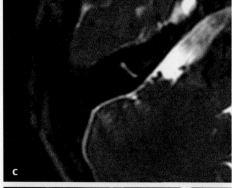

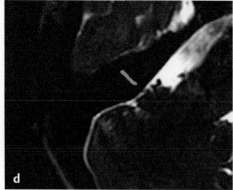

Fig. 3.2 **(a, b)** HRCT temporal bone, axial section, bone window and **(c, d)** MRI CISS/FIESTA axial section show (■ orange) dome of superior semicircular canal (SCC).

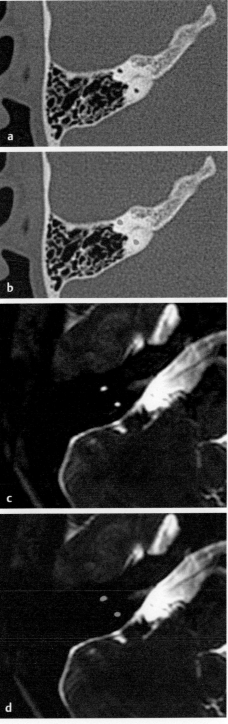

Fig. 3.3 **(a, b)** HRCT temporal bone, axial section, bone window and **(c, d)** MRI CISS/FIESTA axial section show (■ orange) anterior (ampullated) and posterior (nonamputated) limb of superior semicircular canal (SCC).

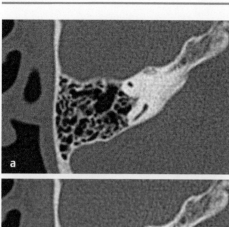

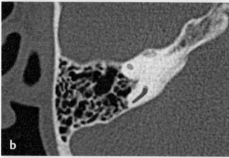

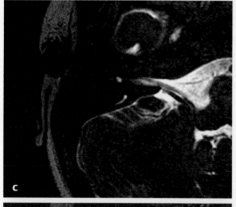

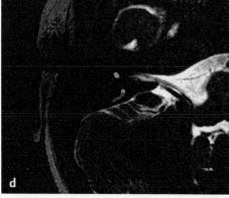

Fig. 3.4 **(a, b)** HRCT temporal bone, axial section, bone window and **(c, d)** MRI CISS/FIESTA axial section show (■ orange) superior semicircular canal (SCC), crus commune (joining of superior SCC and posterior SCC) and (■ pink) posterior SCC.

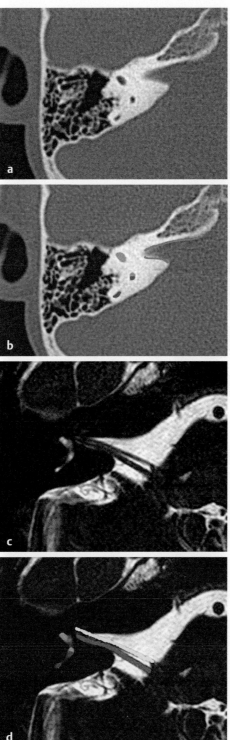

Fig. 3.5 (a, b) HRCT temporal bone, axial section, bone window and **(c, d)** MRI CISS/FIESTA sequence, axial section show (█ orange) superior semicircular canal (SCC), crus commune (joining of superior SCC and posterior SCC), (█ pink) posterior SCC, (yellow) meatal segment of facial nerve, (█ brown) superior vestibular nerve, and (█ green) IAC.

More inferiorly, we will be seeing the various inner ear structures coming into view. If we were to imagine a line running through the long axis of IAC, then the inner ear structures anterior to this line are the cochlear structures and those lying posterior to this line are the vestibular structures. This is especially helpful in many cases of inner ear malformations.

The first structures that we see are (anterior to posterior) the middle turn of the cochlea, the labyrinthine segment of the facial nerve, the superior vestibular nerve, and the vestibule. Here the authors would like to emphasize that the first part of the cochlea which we see in the axial sections, as we go from superior to inferior, is the middle turn and not the apical or the basal turn of the cochlea (**Fig. 3.6**). Just inferiorly (**Fig. 3.7**), we see the "signet ring appearance" or "bucket handle appearance" of the lateral SCC and the vestibule. Also visualized is the vestibular aqueduct, joining the posterior cranial fossa to the vestibule. It is a very narrow structure and may not be seen in many normal HRCT temporal bone scans. Anteriorly, the cochlea gets more well defined. The major content of the vestibular aqueduct is the endolymphatic duct. The MRI at the same level shows the facial nerve (anteriorly) and superior vestibular nerve (posteriorly) in the IAC. MRI will also show the endolymphatic duct and sac. This will be more prominent when endolymphatic duct and sac are dilated. More about this is discussed in the next chapter. Often, a vascular loop is present at the medial end of IAC. In the majority of cases, this is just an incidental finding with no clinical significance. MRI will also show the division between the scala tympani and scala vestibuli of the basal turn of the cochlea by the OSL. The MRI section just inferior shows the cochlear nerve (anteriorly) and inferior vestibular nerve (posteriorly) in the IAC (**Fig. 3.8**); the rest of the structures are pretty similar.

The next section shows better defined turns of cochlea, the modiolus and various septations within the cochlea (**Fig. 3.9**). It also shows the saccule and the tympanic segment of the facial nerve. On the MRI, the same structures are much better defined. The cochlear nerve and inferior vestibular nerve stand out against the contrasting background of the CSF in the IAC. A detailed review of this section is essential because we are able to identify the various inner ear malformations based on the lamina cribrosa, modiolus, septations and cochlear turns, and length.

Modiolus is seen as a hyperdense "crown" shaped structure in the center of the cochlea that gives rise to various septations dividing the cochlea into various turns. It is seen as a hypointense structure in contrast to the bright signal of fluid in the cochlea. For better delineation, CISS/FIESTA images are the best as described in Chapter 1.

In the same section, cochlear aperture can be identified. As described earlier, it is the opening at the fundus of the internal auditory canal through which the eighth nerve enters the cochlea. It is considered to be normal if it is between 1.4 and 3 mm in size.[3] We will be discussing this in detail in Chapter 4 on "Inner Ear Malformations."

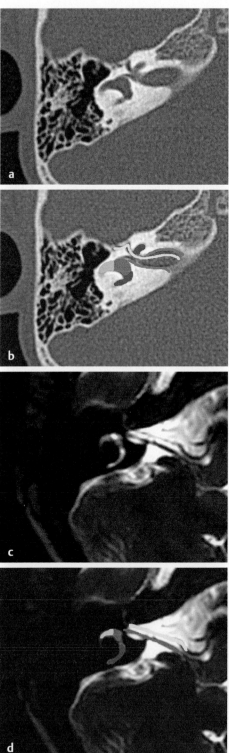

Fig. 3.6 (a, b) HRCT temporal bone, axial section, bone window and **(c, d)** MRI CISS/FIESTA sequence, axial section show (█ pink) posterior semicircular canal (SCC), (yellow) meatal and labyrinthine segment of the facial nerve, (█ dark pink) middle turn of the cochlea, (█ brown) vestibule and superior vestibular nerve, (light green) lateral SCC, and (█ dark green) IAC.

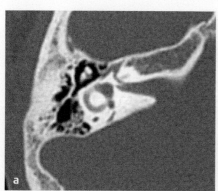

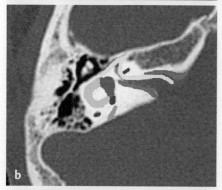

Fig. 3.7 **(a, b)** HRCT temporal bone, axial section, bone window and **(c, d)** MRI CISS/FIESTA sequence, axial section show (■ pink) posterior semicircular canal (SCC), (░ yellow) meatal and labyrinthine segment of the facial nerve, (■ dark pink) middle turn of cochlea, (■ brown) vestibule and superior vestibular nerve, (░ light green) lateral SCC, (░ blue) vestibular aqueduct, and (■ dark green) IAC.

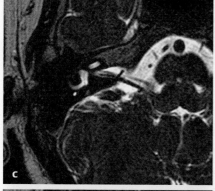

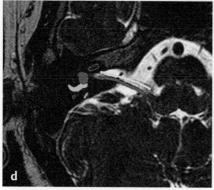

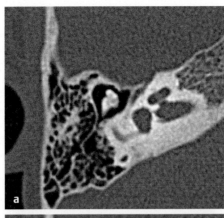

Fig. 3.8 (a, b) HRCT temporal bone, axial section, bone window and **(c, d)** MRI CISS/FIESTA sequence, axial section show (■ pink) posterior semicircular canal (SCC), (□ yellow) tympanic segment of facial nerve, (■ purple) apical turn of cochlea, (■ dark pink) middle turn of cochlea, (■ blue) cochlear nerve, (■ brown) vestibule and inferior vestibular nerve, (□ light green) lateral SCC, (□ light blue) modiolus, and (■ dark green) IAC.

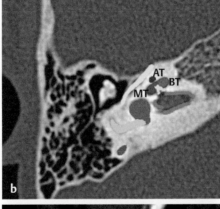

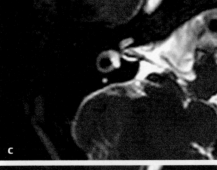

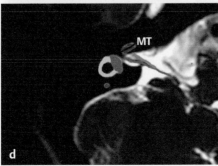

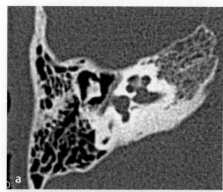

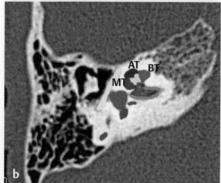

Fig. 3.9 (a, b) HRCT temporal bone, axial section, bone window and **(c, d)** MRI CISS/FIESTA, axial section show (■ pink) posterior semicircular canal (SCC), (▢ yellow) tympanic segment of the facial nerve, (■ purple) apical turn of cochlea, (■ dark pink) middle turn of cochlea, (■ blue) cochlear nerve, (■ brown) vestibule, inferior vestibular nerve and singular nerve (HRCT), (▢ light green) lateral SCC, (▢ light blue) modiolus, (■ dark green) IAC and red arrow shows Rosenthal's canal (RC).

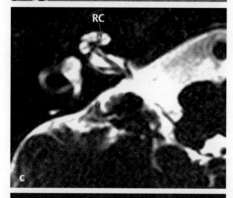

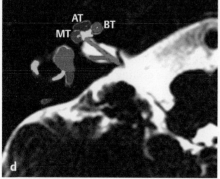

CISS/FIESTA images in MRI would show the Rosenthal's canals travelling in the OSL which carries cochlear nerve fibers and would also show cochlear nerve exiting from the cochlea through the cochlear aperture and entering the IAC. The presence of a cochlear nerve is essential to plan the patient for a cochlear implant. It is better to look for this nerve in oblique sagittals, which will be discussed later in this chapter.

In the next cut, it is important to differentiate between the saccule and the cochlea. The middle and apical turn of cochlea also start taking their shape. One important structure which starts appearing is the cochlear aqueduct. It connects the posterior cranial fossa to the scala tympani of the basal turn of the cochlea, near the round window. From medial to lateral, the IAC has been divided into four segments which consist of medial orifice, otic capsule segment, labyrinthine segment, and lateral orifice. The lateral orifice is the opening into the basal turn of the cochlea, located along the anteroinferior edge of the scala tympani immediately anterior to the crest of the attachment of the round window.[4] The otic capsule segment courses through the labyrinthine bone and never exceeds 2 mm at maximal diameter. The petrous apex segment courses through extralabyrinthine petrous bone, which may or may not be pneumatized, and is more variable in size (average diameter of 4.5 mm). This segment widens as it approaches the funnel-shaped medial orifice which opens into the subarachnoid space adjacent to the jugular foramen.

Cochlear aqueduct is usually patent only in the medial part (medial orifice and otic capsule segment) and closes off as it reaches the cochlea (**Fig. 3.10**). However, it is considered a pathway for the spread of infection from the intracranial region to the cochlea and vice versa. It is considered dilated if it is patent all the way up to the cochlea and can lead to CSF gusher on opening the cochlea during surgery.

There are a few more channels which have an important anatomical and functional role. An accessory cochlear aqueduct (Cotugno's canal) transmits the inferior cochlear vein. This vein terminates within either the inferior petrosal sinus or the jugular bulb. The tympanomeningeal fissure (Hyrtl's fissure), also known as the second accessory canal, develops as a patent communication between the round window and posterior fossa, normally closing at 26 weeks gestation. This structure contains perilymph and, when patent, is much smaller than the cochlear aqueduct. As we will see below, an anomalously patent Hyrtl's fissure is a potential site of congenital CSF otorrhea.

Further inferiorly, the basal, middle, and apical turns become more well-defined and the round window can be visualized well (**Fig. 3.11**). With every cut that we go inferior, the cochlea keeps getting smaller and only the basal turn is now identifiable (**Figs. 3.12** and **3.13**). After cochlea finishes, only the internal carotid artery and jugular bulb are identifiable (**Fig. 3.14**).

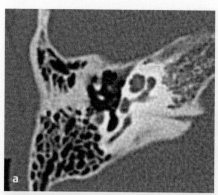

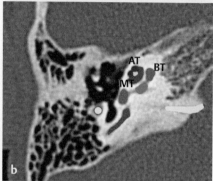

Fig. 3.10 (a, b) HRCT temporal bone, axial section, bone window and **(c, d)** MRI CISS/FIESTA sequence, axial section show (■ pink) posterior semicircular canal (SCC), (□ yellow) mastoid segment of facial nerve, (■ purple) apical turn of cochlea, (■ dark pink) middle turn of cochlea, (■ brown) vestibule, (□ light blue) modiolus, (■ dark green) IAC, and (□ light yellow) cochlear aqueduct.

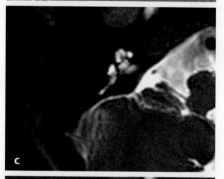

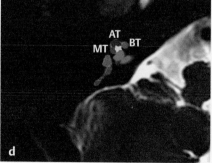

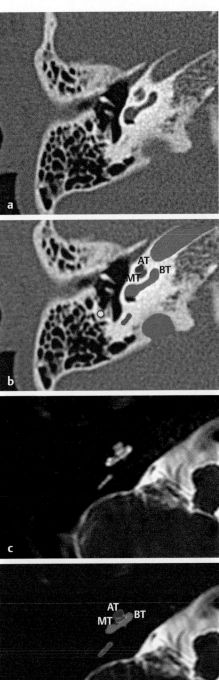

Fig. 3.11 (a, b) HRCT temporal bone, axial section, bone window and **(c, d)** MRI CISS/FIESTA sequence, axial section show (■ pink) posterior semicircular canal, (□ yellow) mastoid segment of the facial nerve, (■ purple) apical turn of the cochlea, (■ dark pink) middle turn of cochlea, (■ dark blue) jugular bulb, and (■ red) internal carotid artery.

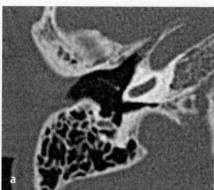

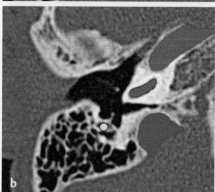

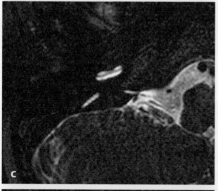

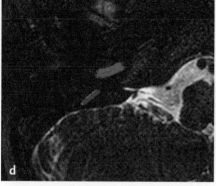

Fig. 3.12 **(a, b)** HRCT temporal bone, axial section, bone window and **(c, d)** MRI CISS/FIESTA sequence, axial section show (■ pink) posterior semicircular canal, (yellow) mastoid segment of the facial nerve, (■ dark blue) jugular bulb, and (■ red) internal carotid artery.

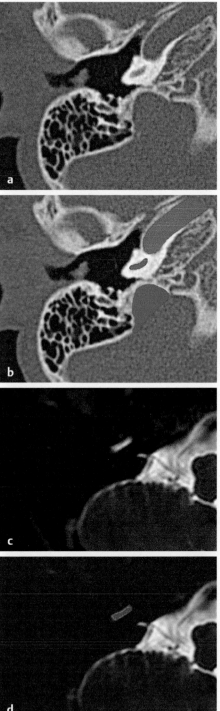

Fig. 3.13 **(a, b)** HRCT temporal bone, axial section, bone window and **(c, d)** MRI CISS/FIESTA sequence, axial section show (☐ yellow) mastoid segment of the facial nerve, (■ dark blue) jugular bulb, and (▨ red) internal carotid artery.

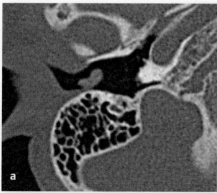

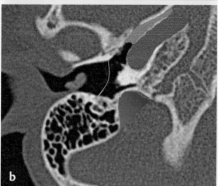

Fig. 3.14 (a, b) HRCT temporal bone, axial section, bone window shows (■ light violet) tympanic membrane, (■ light brown) eustachian tube, (■ dark blue) jugular bulb, and (■ red) internal carotid artery.

Coronal Sections

The coronal sections are by convention read from anterior to posterior. The most anterior structure is the internal carotid artery (**Fig. 3.15**). As we go posterior, we start seeing various sections of the cochlea and the facial nerve (**Figs. 3.16, 3.17, 3.18,** and **3.19**). These relations are very important as the cochlea–carotid interval can be very less and sometimes there might be no bone between the two.[5] Surgeons have put electrodes in the carotid canal due to this proximity and lack of knowledge of anatomy and radiology. Similarly, the labyrinthine segment of the facial nerve is very close to the middle turn of cochlea and there have been cases of facial nerve stimulation especially in patients with otosclerosis. The nerves in the IAC can be visualized in coronal sections too; however, it is not easy to differentiate between these nerves.

As we go more posterior, we start seeing the vestibule and the lateral and superior SCCs (**Figs. 3.20, 3.21, 3.22,** and **3.23**) and then the oval and round windows. In the section, where lateral and superior SCCs are seen as dots and vestibule as a bigger dot, the authors like to call that as the Mickey Mouse sign (**Fig. 3.22**).

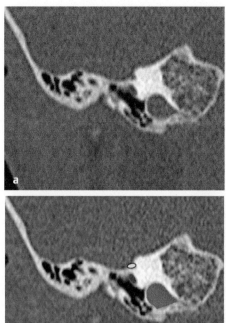

Fig. 3.15 (a, b) HRCT temporal bone, coronal section, bone window shows (yellow) geniculate ganglion of the facial nerve, (■ dark brown) tensor tympani, and (■ red) internal carotid artery.

In the posterior most sections, we can see the posterior SCC and the vestibular aqueduct (**Figs. 3.24** and **3.25**). This is important because we can compare the dimensions of the endolymphatic duct with that of the posterior SCC to find out if the former is dilated. We will be discussing this more in the chapter on inner ear malformations.

Imaging the IAC: Oblique Sagittal Sections (Stenver's Projection) of T2 MRI

These are very important sections in MRI as they help us identify the cochlear nerve and its anomalies in the best possible manner. Multiple oblique sagittal sections of the IAC are taken in CISS/FIESTA MRI sequence. These sections show the vestibulocochlear and facial nerves arising from the cerebellopontine angle (CP angle) and going to the inner ear. It is important to remember that by looking at one section we cannot tell whether it is of the right side or the left side. For this, it is important to see the scout film and remember that these sections go from lateral to medial on one side and then medial to lateral on the other side. So both the sides look exactly similar and are not lateral inversions of each other.

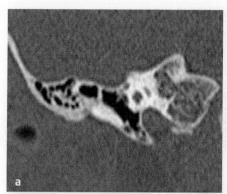

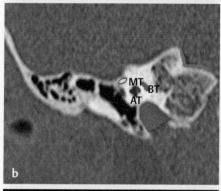

Fig. **(a, b)** HRCT temporal bone, coronal section, bone window and **(c, d)** MRI CISS/FIESTA sequence show (■ purple) apical turn of the cochlea, (■ dark pink) middle turn of the cochlea, (☐ yellow) labyrinthine segment of the facial nerve, (■ dark green) IAC, and (■ red) internal carotid artery.

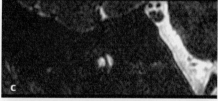

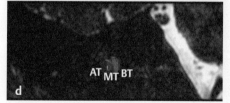

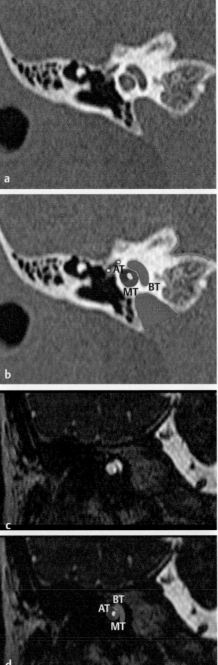

Fig. 3.17 **(a, b)** HRCT temporal bone, coronal section, bone window and **(c, d)** MRI CISS/FIESTA sequence show (■ purple) apical turn of the cochlea, (■ dark pink) middle turn of the cochlea, (■ light blue) modiolus, (■ dark green) IAC, (yellow) tympanic and labyrinthine segment of the facial nerve (snake eye appearance), and (■ red) internal carotid artery.

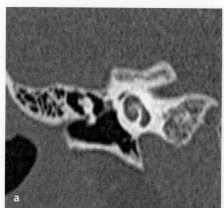

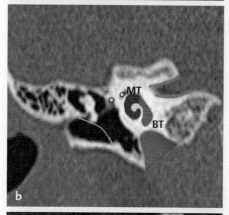

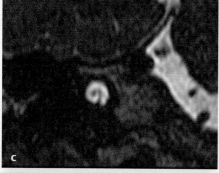

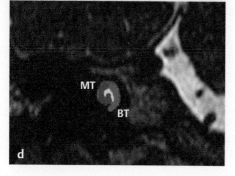

Fig. 3.18 **(a, b)** HRCT temporal bone, coronal section, bone window and **(c, d)** MRI CISS/FIESTA, sequence show (█ purple) apical turn of the cochlea, (█ dark pink) middle turn of the cochlea, (█ light pink) basal turn of cochlea, (█ light blue) modiolus, (█ dark green) IAC, (█ yellow) tympanic and labyrinthine segment of the facial nerve (snake eye appearance), and (█ red) internal carotid artery.

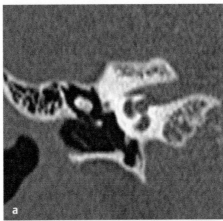

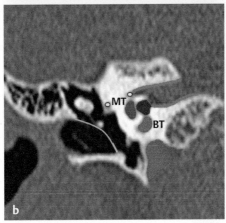

Fig. 3.19 (a, b) HRCT temporal bone, coronal section, bone window shows (■ light pink) basal turn of cochlea, (■ dark pink) middle turn of the cochlea, (■ brown) vestibule, (■ dark green) IAC, (■ yellow) tympanic and labyrinthine segment of the facial nerve (snake eye appearance), and (■ red) internal carotid artery.

As we go from medial to lateral, initially only the facial nerve and the vestibulocochlear nerve complex are seen (**Fig. 3.26**). The latter has not differentiated into various nerves. Normally, the vestibulocochlear nerve complex at this level is more than twice the width of the facial nerve. In the next section, we see the facial nerve and the vestibulocochlear nerve complex entering the IAC (**Fig. 3.27**). So, at the level of CP angle, also referred to as the porus of the IAC, we see only two dots: the facial nerve and the vestibulocochlear nerve complex.

As we reach the level of the middle part of the IAC, we start seeing three dots: the facial nerve, the vestibular nerve, and the cochlear nerve (**Figs. 3.28** and **3.29**). The vestibular nerve has not differentiated into the superior and inferior vestibular nerve yet.

Going more medially, as we reach the fundus of the IAC, we start seeing four dots: the facial and superior vestibular nerves in the superior half, and the cochlear and the inferior vestibular nerves in the inferior half (**Figs. 3.30** and **3.31**). In the most medial sections, we see the cochlear nerve entering the modiolus of the cochlea (**Fig. 3.32**).

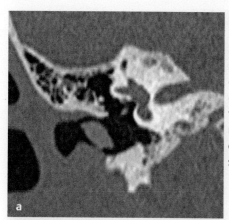

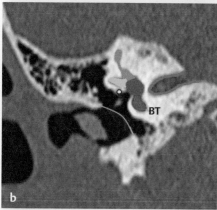

Fig. 3.20 (a, b) HRCT temporal bone, coronal section, bone window and **(c, d)** MRI CISS/FIESTA sequence show (■ light pink) basal turn of cochlea, (■ brown) vestibule, (■ dark green) IAC, (yellow) tympanic segment of the facial nerve, (■ light green) lateral semicircular canal (SCC), and (■ orange) superior SCC.

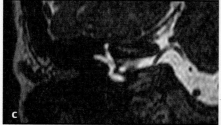

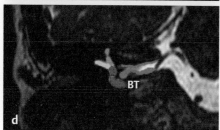

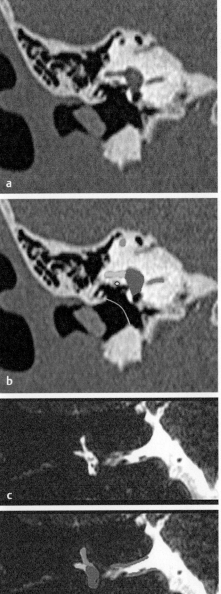

Fig. 3.21 (a, b) HRCT temporal bone, coronal section, bone window and **(c, d)** MRI CISS/FIESTA sequence show (■ brown) vestibule, (■ dark green) IAC, (□ yellow) tympanic segment of facial nerve, (□ light green) lateral semicircular canal (SCC), and (■ orange) superior SCC.

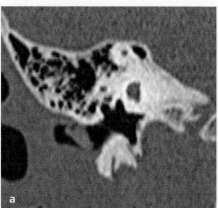

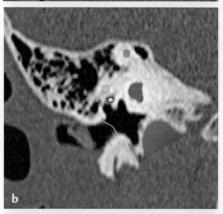

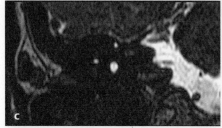

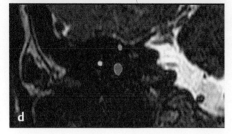

Fig. 3.22 (a, b) HRCT temporal bone, coronal section, bone window and **(c, d)** MRI CISS/FIESTA sequence show (yellow) tympanic segment of the facial nerve, (█ brown) vestibule, (light green) lateral semicircular canal (SCC), (█ orange) superior SCC, and (█ dark blue) jugular bulb. Mickey Mouse sign (the lateral and superior semicircular canals and the vestibule) is also seen.

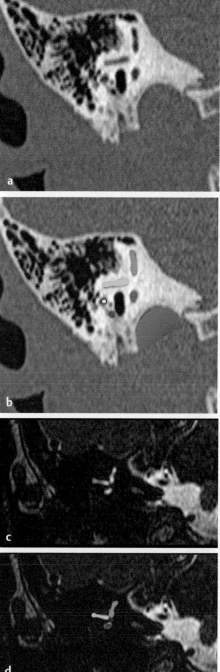

Fig. 3.23 **(a, b)** HRCT temporal bone, coronal section, bone window and **(c, d)** MRI CISS/FIESTA sequence show (■ brown) vestibule, (　yellow) tympanic segment of facial nerve, (　light green) lateral semicircular canal (SCC), (■ pink) posterior SCC, (■ orange) superior SCC, and (■ dark blue) jugular bulb.

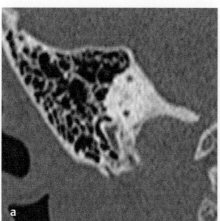

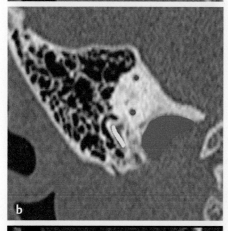

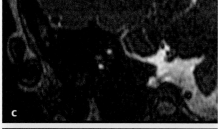

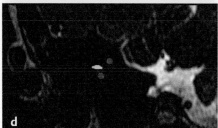

Fig. 3.24 (a, b) HRCT temporal bone, coronal section, bone window and **(c, d)** MRI CISS/FIESTA sequence show (yellow) mastoid segment of facial nerve, (light green) lateral semicircular canal (SCC), (pink) posterior SCC, and (dark blue) jugular bulb.

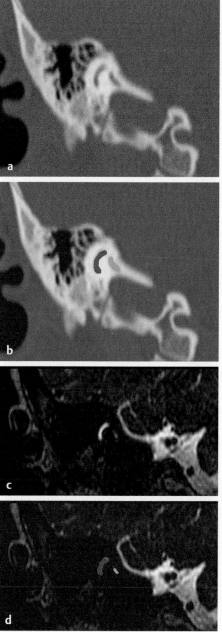

Fig. 3.25 **(a, b)** HRCT temporal bone, coronal section, bone window and **(c, d)** MRI CISS/FIESTA sequence show (■ pink) posterior semicircular canal and (■ blue) vestibular aqueduct.

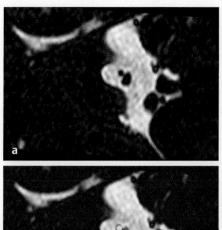

Fig. 3.26 (a, b) MRI CISS/ FIESTA sequence, oblique sagittal reformation images at the level of CP angle show (yellow) facial nerve and (■ brown) vestibulocochlear nerve complex.

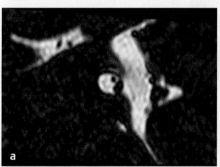

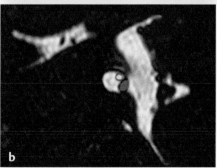

Fig. 3.27 (a, b) MRI CISS/ FIESTA sequence, oblique sagittal reformation images at the level of porus of IAC show (yellow) facial nerve and (■ brown) vestibulocochlear nerve complex.

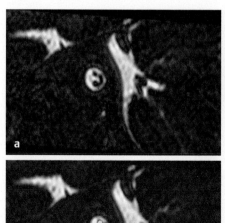

Fig. 3.28 (a, b) MRI CISS/ FIESTA sequence, oblique sagittal reformation images at mid part of IAC show (yellow) facial nerve, (brown) vestibular nerve, and (blue) cochlear nerve.

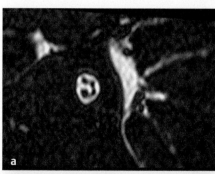

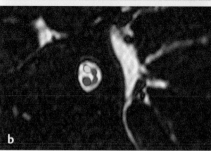

Fig. 3.29 (a, b) MRI CISS/ FIESTA sequence, oblique sagittal reformation images at mid part of IAC show (yellow) facial nerve and (brown) vestibular nerve, and (blue) cochlear nerve.

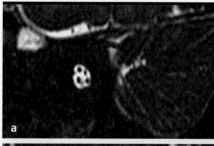

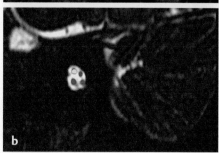

Fig. 3.30 (a, b) MRI CISS/ FIESTA sequence, oblique sagittal reformation images at fundus of IAC show (yellow) facial nerve, (█ brown) superior vestibular nerve above and inferior vestibular nerve below, and (█ blue) cochlear nerve.

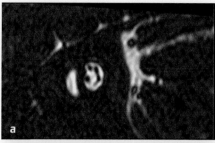

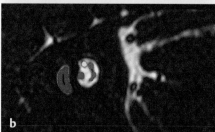

Fig. 3.31 (a, b) MRI CISS/ FIESTA sequence, oblique sagittal reformation at the fundus of IAC shows (yellow) facial nerve, (█ brown) superior vestibular nerve above and inferior vestibular nerve below with singular nerve, (█ dark pink) cochlea, and (█ blue) cochlear nerve.

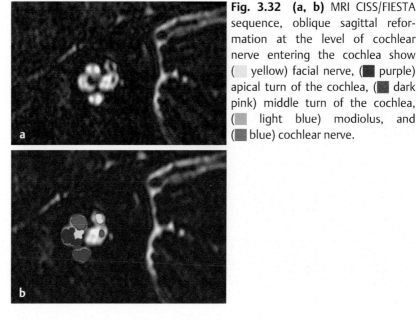

Fig. 3.32 (a, b) MRI CISS/FIESTA sequence, oblique sagittal reformation at the level of cochlear nerve entering the cochlea show (yellow) facial nerve, (■ purple) apical turn of the cochlea, (■ dark pink) middle turn of the cochlea, (light blue) modiolus, and (■ blue) cochlear nerve.

Oblique Sagittal Images (Stenver's Projection) of the Cochlea

These images are good to understand the "hook" region of the cochlea. As discussed in the previous chapter, oblique sagittal reconstructions of the HRCT temporal bones give a good view of the basal and middle turn of the cochlea, facial nerve, oval window, and round window (**Fig. 3.33**). With the recent literature supporting round window insertions, round window has become the preferred site for entry into the cochlea in many centers. However, technically electrode insertion through the round window is more difficult primarily due to the "hook" region. The "hook" region is defined as the most basal part of the cochlea which forms a fish hook–like curvature in three dimensions.[6,7] This portion contains the cul-de-sac of the endolymphatic space where the OSL, spiral ligament, and basilar membrane merge. Surgical problem with this area is that the acute angulation may lead to difficulty in electrode insertion. Let us try to understand it with help of these hypothetical radiology pictures. In order to do round window insertion, the first thing which is done is drilling the round window niche (**Fig. 3.34**). Then the round window is incised and the electrodes are inserted. The round window is not in direct line with the axis of the lumen of the basal turn of the scala tympani. So when we insert the electrodes from the round window, they might hit the OSL and then get deflected toward the desired lumen. In a simple language, there is a significant angulation which may need to be overcome during electrode

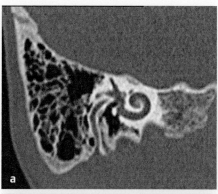

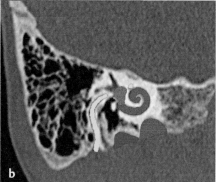

Fig. 3.33 (a, b) HRCT temporal bone, oblique sagittal reconstruction, bone window shows (yellow) labyrinthine, tympanic, second genu, and mastoid segment of the facial nerve; (dark pink) cochlea; (red) internal carotid artery; (dark blue) jugular bulb; (light blue) stapes at oval window; (light brown) saccule; and (white arrow) round window.

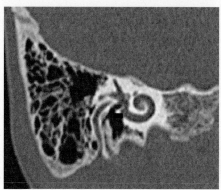

Fig. 3.34 HRCT temporal bone, oblique sagittal reconstruction, bone window shows the way round window is exposed after drilling the niche.

insertion (**Fig. 3.35a**). This angulation may vary from patient to patient. One of the ways to overcome this angulation is to drill the crista fenestra. In case of unfavorable anatomy, the angulation may be very acute and complete insertion may not be possible. Such patients require separate cochleostomy. Separate cochleostomy usually gives good access into the basal turn (**Fig. 3.35b**); however, the inherent issues with drilling the bone are there.

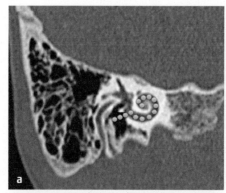

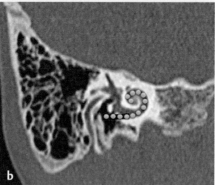

Fig. 3.35 HRCT temporal bone, oblique sagittal reconstruction, bone window shows schematic representation of the electrodes inserted through **(a)** round window approach and the effect an adverse "hook" region may have and **(b)** electrode inserted through separate cochleostomy, in line with the axis of basal turn. "Hook" region may therefore create difficulty in electrode insertion and needs to be dealt with properly during surgery.

Cochlear Duct Length

Over the past few years, there has been a renewed interest in the anatomy of the cochlea. There have been various articles on cochlear duct length and all of them have found that the length of cochlea varies from person to person. Many authors are of the view that because of this variation, electrode arrays of individualized lengths should be used as per the length of the cochlea of that particular patient. Historically, many methods have been used to calculate the length of the cochlea. One of the most initial methods was by direct measurement under histopathology with a micrometer.[8] Since then, various other direct and indirect methodologies have been used for this purpose. Recently, the majority of studies use radiology and mathematical equations to find out cochlear duct length. One of the major studies in this regard was done by Alexiades et al in Europe and North America.[9] Using the same method, Grover et al did a study in the Asian population and found the values to range from 28 to 34.3 mm (mean 29.8 mm).[10] They concluded that probably the cochlea is shorter in the Asian population. In both these studies, the formula used to calculate this was CDL = 4.16A – 3.98, where CDL is cochlear duct length and A is the measured largest distance from the round window to the lateral wall of cochlea passing through modiolus in oblique sagittal reconstruction of the cochlea (**Fig. 3.36a**). The other way to calculate A is by measuring the distance between the round window and farthest point on the basal turn in the axial section (**Fig. 3.36b**).

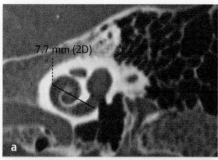

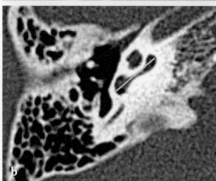

Fig. 3.36 HRCT temporal bone window shows, **(a)** measurement of variable *A* in oblique sagittal reconstruction section, **(b)** measurement of variable *A* in axial section.

Authors believe that its impact on hearing outcomes are yet to be proven; however, it may definitely injure a shorter cochlea and cause tip roll overs in a longer cochlea specially if a modiolus hugging electrode is being used. In general it has been agreed that the minimum length of a normal cochlea is 25 mm. This is discussed more in the chapter on inner ear malformations.

Cochlear Orientation

Visualization of the round window from posterior tympanotomy is variable. In some patients, we have the full round window visualized very well. On the other extreme, there are patients where we cannot even see the round window after an optimum posterior tympanotomy. St Thomas classification is based on the same:[11]

- Type I: 100% visualization of round window.
- Type IIa: 50 to 99% visualization of round window.
- Type IIb: 1 to 49% visualization of round window.
- Type III: Round window not visualized.

This could be due to various reasons such as facial recess width, obliquity of external auditory canal, and cochlear orientation. Cochlea can be oriented (rotated) anteriorly or posteriorly. In the case of posterior orientation, the round window is more posteriorly oriented and therefore hidden under the facial nerve. This makes it difficult for it to be visualized. The other problem which is faced with the more posteriorly rotated cochlea is the angulation which is encountered during electrode insertion. This makes round window insertion more difficult. Grover et al calculated this orientation by calculating the angle between midsagittal plane and long axis of the basal turn of cochlea in the axial section (**Fig. 3.37**).[12] They found out that this orientation was variable and different even on either side (**Fig. 3.38**). They concluded that whenever this angle (which they called as α) was less than 50 degrees, the operating surgeon had difficulty in electrode insertion.[12]

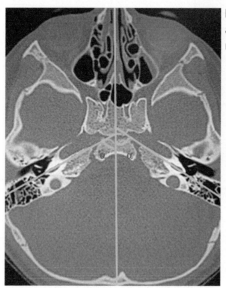

Fig. 3.37 HRCT temporal bone, axial section, bone window showing measurement of angle α.

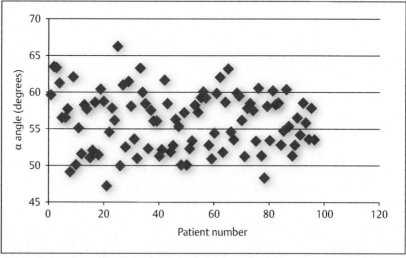

Fig. 3.38 Scatter diagram showing the value of angle α in the study done by Grover et al.[12]

Cochlear Cleft

It is a variable area of incomplete ossification in the otic capsule just adjacent to the cochlea, present usually in children. It is a curvilinear C-shaped radiolucent structure present lateral to the basal turn of the cochlea, just anterior to the oval window (**Fig. 3.39**). It is not so commonly seen in adults and many times a focus of otosclerosis may be confused with the cochlear cleft. However, it should be remembered that fissula ante fenestram is posterior to the site of the cochlear cleft. The cochlear cleft is a normal variant seen in up to 40% of the pediatric population and has no bearing whatsoever on hearing loss.[13]

3D Reconstruction of Inner Ear

With the help of software on CT machines, the inner ear can be reconstructed to better understand the anatomy. This is especially useful in cases with cochleovestibular malformations and ossification. **Fig. 3.40** shows 3D reconstruction of the normal inner ear on HRCT temporal bone. This can also be used for teaching purposes.

Recent Advances

Robotic Cochlear Implant

With the first robotic cochlear implant being done in Switzerland,[14] authors are sure that with time it will become more popular. One of the most important pillars for this would be radiology as it helps decide the surgical plan. Four surgical fiducial screws, for patient to image registration, are implanted into the mastoid. The software defines and calculates various things (**Fig. 3.41**). These include the part of the chorda tympani in the middle ear, the site of proposed entry into the cochlea, the drilling angle, and the distances from the tunnel to the surrounding important anatomical structures. All this is important to prevent any catastrophic complications.

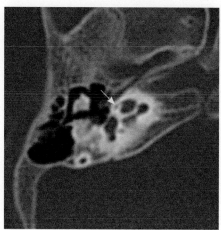

Fig. 3.39 HRCT temporal bone window, axial section shows cochlear cleft (yellow arrow).

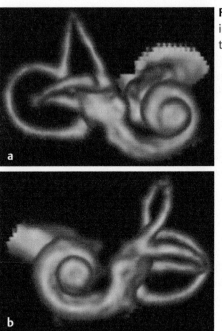

Fig. 3.40 (a, b) 3D reconstructed images of the inner ear on HRCT temporal bone.

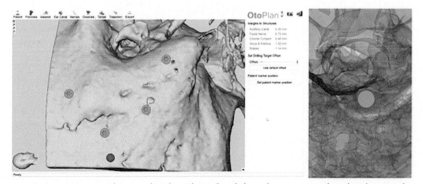

Fig. 3.41 Green color marks the place for fiducial screws and red color marks the bone anchored dynamic reference base marker. The planned access to the cochlea (blue), the facial nerve (yellow), the chorda tympani (orange), the ear canal wall (dark blue), and the ossicles (violet) are thereby marked with the help of software.[14]

References

1.   Valvassori GE, Clemis JD. The large vestibular aqueduct syndrome. Laryngoscope 1978;88(5):723–728
2.   Wilson DF, Hodgson RS, Talbot JM. Endolymphatic sac obliteration for large vestibular aqueduct syndrome. Am J Otol 1997;18(1):101–106, discussion 106–107
3.   Stjernholm C, Muren C. Dimensions of the cochlear nerve canal: a radioanatomic investigation. Acta Otolaryngol 2002;122(1):43–48
4.   Jackler RK, Hwang PH. Enlargement of the cochlear aqueduct: fact or fiction? Otolaryngol Head Neck Surg 1993;109(1):14–25
5.   Young RJ, Shatzkes DR, Babb JS, Lalwani AK. The cochlear-carotid interval: anatomic variation and potential clinical implications. AJNR Am J Neuroradiol 2006;27(7):1486–1490
6.   Stidham KR, Roberson JB Jr. Cochlear hook anatomy: evaluation of the spatial relationship of the basal cochlear duct to middle ear landmarks. Acta Otolaryngol 1999;119(7):773–777
7.   Li PM, Wang H, Northrop C, Merchant SN, Nadol JB Jr. Anatomy of the round window and hook region of the cochlea with implications for cochlear implantation and other endocochlear surgical procedures. Otol Neurotol 2007;28(5):641–648
8.   Hardy M. The length of the organ of Corti in man. Am J Anat 1938;62(2):291–311
9.   Alexiades G, Dhanasingh A, Jolly C. Method to estimate the complete and two-turn cochlear duct length. Otol Neurotol 2015;36(5):904–907
10. Grover M, Sharma S, Singh SN, Kataria T, Lakhawat RS, Sharma MP. Measuring cochlear duct length in Asian population: worth giving a thought! Eur Arch Otorhinolaryngol 2018;275(3):725–728
11. Leong AC, Jiang D, Agger A, Fitzgerald-O'Connor A. Evaluation of round window accessibility to cochlear implant insertion. Eur Arch Otorhinolaryngol 2013;270(4):1237–1242
12. Sharma S, Grover M, Singh SN, Kataria T, Lakhawat RS. Cochlear orientation: pre-operative evaluation and intra-operative significance. J Laryngol Otol 2018;132(6):540–543
13. Chadwell JB, Halsted MJ, Choo DI, Greinwald JH, Benton C. The cochlear cleft. AJNR Am J Neuroradiol 2004;25(1):21–24
14. Caversaccio M, Gavaghan K, Wimmer W, et al. Robotic cochlear implantation: surgical procedure and first clinical experience. Acta Otolaryngol 2017;137(4):447–454

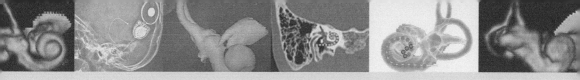

Chapter 4

Inner Ear Malformations

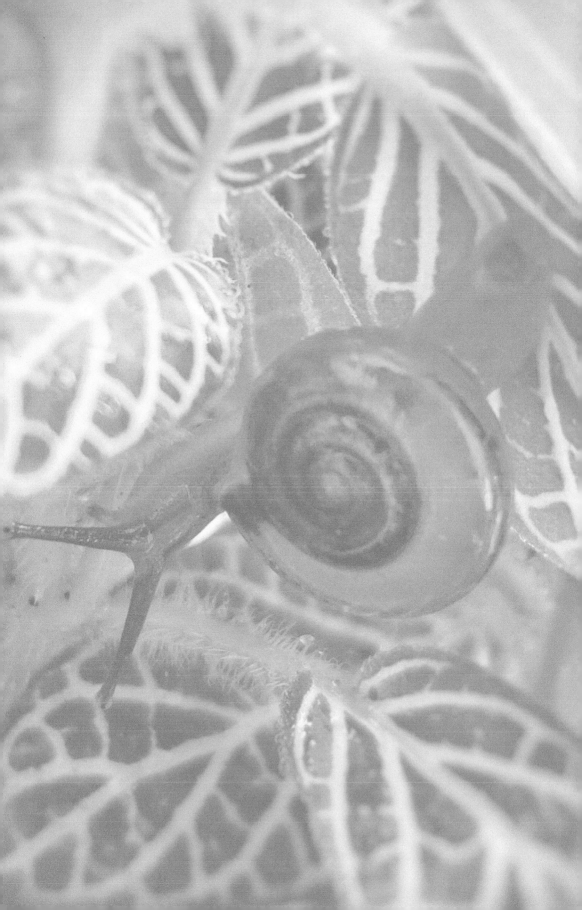

4 Inner Ear Malformations

Introduction

With the advent of technology, cochlear implantation has become the standard treatment for patients with bilateral severe-to-profound sensorineural hearing loss. Suitable candidates provide us with gratifying results; however, when a patient has poor results, it can be upsetting for the patient and the surgeon. Cochleovestibular malformation is one preoperative predictor of outcome. Inner ear malformations are found in 10 to 30% of patients with congenital sensorineural deafness on high-resolution computed tomography (HRCT) of the temporal bone[1,2] made possible with advances in imaging. Identifying these malformations is important preoperatively as it has a significant impact on surgical technique, electrode array choice, surgical complications, and cochlear implantation results.[3] Therefore, proper consent is also needed.

Embryology

Knowledge regarding the embryogenesis of the inner ear is important to understand the development of various inner ear malformations. During the third week of gestation, there is thickening of the surface ectoderm on either side of the rhombencephalon, resulting in an otic placode. The otic placode invaginates to form an otic pit. Around fourth week the otic pit closes off to form an otocyst. During the fifth week, the labyrinth is well-differentiated into vestibular and cochlear pouches. Vestibular portion forms first which is followed by the cochlear portion development. By sixth week, the anterior pouch of labyrinth elongates to form the cochlea. Cochlea attains adult size by 10 weeks of gestation. Differentiation of organ of Corti starts by 10th week and cochlea is fully developed by sixth month. The labyrinth is fully formed by 5 months of gestation. The ganglion cells of the vestibulocochlear nerve arise from the otic vesicle during the fourth week and all synapses both afferent and efferent are formed by the seventh fetal month. The maturation of connections between the cochlea and peripheral nerves takes place during the last trimester. The internal acoustic canal (IAC) is formed by inhibition of cartilage formation at the medial aspect of the otic vesicle. This presence of the vestibulocochlear nerve is required for this inhibition to occur. In the absence of the eighth nerve, IAC is not formed.

History of Classifications

In 1791, Carlo Mondini (1729–1803), dissected the temporal bone of an 8-year-old boy who was deaf. The child had an accident with a carriage, leading to foot infection and later gangrene. In those days, as there were no antibiotics the boy succumbed to this infection. Mondini dissected his temporal bone and identified three things, viz superior coil of the cochlea was missing, the entire labyrinth was enlarged, and the vestibular aqueduct (VA) was very large. This triad thus came to be known as Mondini's dysplasia. Sadly for the next two centuries, almost every malformation of the inner ear was labelled as Mondini's dysplasia.[4] After renewed interest in the inner ear due to cochlear implants (CIs), various classifications for cochleovestibular malformations were put forward. The accepted ones include those of Jackler et al (1987),[1] Phelps et al (1992),[5] Sennaroğlu et al (2002),[6] and Grover et al (2019).[7] Prior to these classifications, almost all malformations were labelled as Mondini's dysplasia. Jackler et al outlined the terms used for malformations as: complete labyrinthine aplasia (CLA), cochlear aplasia (CA), cochlear hypoplasia (CH), incomplete partition (IP), and common cavity (CC). However, as there was no detailed description of the terms and as it was based on the development of the inner ear, the clinical significance of this classification gradually declined. Other classifications could not gain much popularity till, in 2002, Sennaroğlu came out with a classification and presently this is the most well accepted classification world over. However authors believe that it is too complex and tough to follow and therefore lacks uniformity. It is not easy for the user to follow and does not predict the prognosis and complications in a graded manner. For these reasons, the authors believe that the Sawai Man Singh (SMS) classification is more practical and will be discussed in detail later. However, the reader should remember that at present, the classification given by Sennaroğlu is the most accepted one worldwide.

Sennaroglu Classification

Sennaroglu came out with multiple papers regarding classification of inner ear malformations.[3,6,8,9,10,11] He has explained the various terminologies used in these malformations in detail, including their histopathology and development. Authors would be discussing each one of them separately in this chapter.

Enlarged Vestibular Aqueduct

One of the most common inner ear malformations is enlarged vestibular aqueduct (EVA). We read in the previous chapter how to identify a normal VA (**Figs. 4.1** and **4.2**). VA is a bony structure which contains the endolymphatic duct which connects the inner ear to the endolymphatic sac in the posterior cranial fossa.

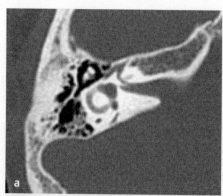

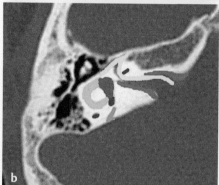

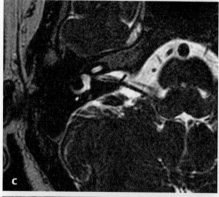

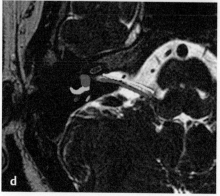

Fig. 4.1 (a, b) HRCT temporal bone, axial section, bone window and **(c, d)** MRI CISS/FIESTA sequence, axial section show (■ pink) posterior semicircular canal (SCC), (☐ yellow) meatal and labyrinthine segment of facial nerve, (■ dark pink) middle turn of cochlea, (■ brown) vestibule and superior vestibular nerve, (☐ light green) lateral SCC, (■ blue) vestibular aqueduct, and (■ dark green) IAC.

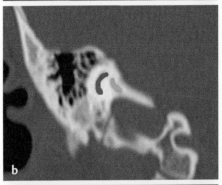

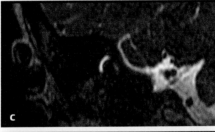

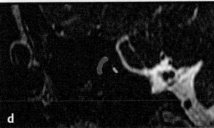

Fig. 4.2 (a, b) HRCT temporal bone, coronal section, bone window and **(c, d)** MRI CISS/FIESTA sequence show (■ pink) posterior semicircular canal, (■ blue) vestibular aqueduct.

Various criteria have been stated for EVA (**Fig. 4.3**); the most common ones which gained acceptance are Valvassori and Clemis criteria, Cincinnati criteria, and Wilson criteria.

1. Valvassori and Clemis criteria (1978): This is the most accepted criteria for the diagnosis of EVA. According to this VA is said to be enlarged if the width measured at the midpoint of its course from the vestibule to the opening (operculum) in the posterior cranial fossa is more than 1.5 mm[12] (**Fig. 4.4**).
2. Cincinnati criteria: In 2007, Boston et al suggested the Cincinnati criteria.[13] They stated that VA is to be considered enlarged if the width measured at the midpoint is greater than 0.9 mm or at the operculum is greater than 1.9 mm.
3. Wilson criteria: Urman and Talbot defined EVA as any segment of the VA twice that of the adjacent posterior semicircular canal (SCC).[14]

EVA can be a sign of a genetic disorder called Pendred syndrome, a cause of childhood hearing loss. Hearing loss associated with Pendred syndrome is usually progressive, which means that a child will lose hearing over time. Another feature of Pendred syndrome is goiter.

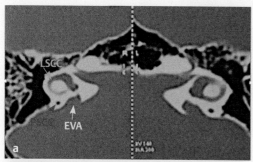
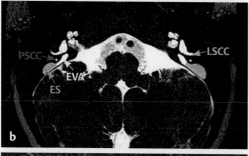
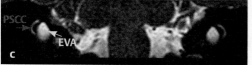

Fig. 4.3 **(a)** HRCT temporal bone, axial section bone window and **(b, c)** MRI CISS sequence, axial and coronal sections show PSCC (pink arrow), LSCC (blue arrow), endolymphatic sac (ES, green arrow) and enlarged vestibular aqueduct (EVA, yellow arrow).

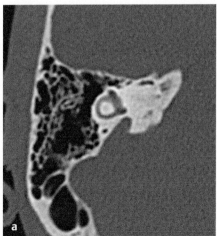

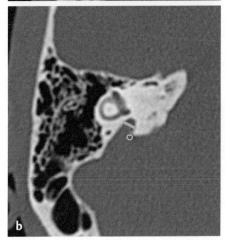

Fig. 4.4 (a, b) HRCT temporal bone, axial section, bone window showing measurement of the width of vestibular aqueduct at the midpoint (blue line) and at operculum (yellow O).

EVA has many causes, not all of which are fully understood. The most well-known cause of EVA and hearing loss is mutations in a gene called *SLC26A4* (previously known as the *PDS* gene). Two mutations in the *SLC26A4* gene can result in Pendred syndrome.

There are two major hypotheses for hearing loss in EVA. The first hypothesis was based on pressure transmission. Repeated minor head trauma could lead to progressive hearing loss due to transmission of the pressure change to the inner ear.[15] This was also proven radiologically by Sennaroglu in a case report where he showed dilatation of scala vestibuli alone in a case of EVA in magnetic resonance imaging (MRI) thereby strengthening the hypothesis that pressure transmission from EVA led to this dilation.[16] However, the majority of recent literature supports the hypothesis that EVA is like a marker to genetic mutation in the *SLC26A4* gene, and the mutation itself is responsible for hearing loss. Grover wrote a letter to the editor in the same respect.[17]

Complete Labyrinthine Aplasia

CLA is also known as Michel deformity. It indicates the absence of any labyrinthine structure. This happens when developmental arrest happens before the formation of otocyst. This is an absolute contraindication for CIs and patients with CLA need auditory brainstem implants. Based on radiological findings, Sennaroglu divided CLA into three types.

CLA with Petrous Bone Aplasia or Hypoplasia

This is seen when CLA is accompanied with absent or minimally developed petrous bone. In such a condition, many times dura may be seen adjacent to the middle ear (**Fig. 4.5**).

CLA without Otic Capsule

In this condition, the inner ear structures are absent however the petrous bone is normally developed (**Fig. 4.6**).

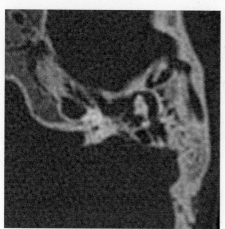

Fig. 4.5 HRCT temporal bone, axial sections, bone window shows CLA with aplastic or hypoplastic petrous bone thereby no inner ear structures are visualized and dura is seen right next to the middle ear.

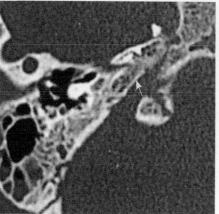

Fig. 4.6 HRCT temporal bone, axial section, bone window shows CLA without otic capsule with presence of petrous bone (yellow arrow).

CLA with Otic Capsule

In this case, the inner ear is completely absent however the otic capsule is developed and therefore we can see the facial nerve running a normal course (**Fig. 4.7**).

Rudimentary Otocyst/Primitive Otocyst (Michel's Otocyst Deformity)

A rudimentary otocyst (RO) (**Fig. 4.8**) is defined as an incomplete millimetric representation of the otic capsule (round or ovoid in shape) without an IAC.[3] The RO occurs due to the developmental arrest between the third and fourth weeks of inner ear embryogenesis. This insult usually occurs at the beginning of the formation of the otocyst. Occasionally, RO can be accompanied by rudimentary SCC formations. RO represents an anomaly between CLA (where there is no inner development) and CC. RO is a very small cystic structure without the formation of IAC. The only option of hearing rehabilitation in RO is by auditory brainstem implants.

Cochlear Aplasia

Important features of CA include:

1. Absence of cochlea.
2. The labyrinthine segment of the facial nerve is displaced anteriorly and occupies the normal location of the cochlea.
3. Vestibule and SCCs occupy their normal anatomic location in the posterolateral part of the fundus of the IAC.
4. The cochlear nerve is absent.

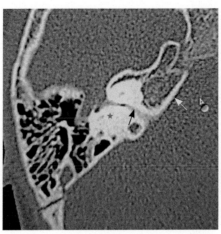

Fig. 4.7 HRCT temporal bone, axial section bone window shows CLA with otic capsule (red star, otic capsule; yellow arrow, petrous bone; black arrow, facial nerve).

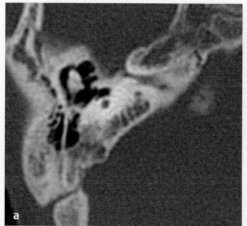

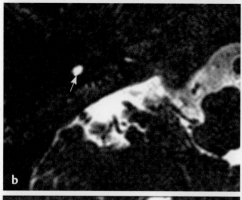

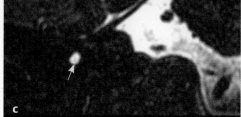

Fig. 4.8 (a) HRCT temporal bone, axial section bone window and **(b)** axial section and **(c)** coronal sections on MRI, CISS sequence show RO (yellow arrow) without internal acoustic canal.

Based on these, if the vestibular system is dilated or not, CA is divided into: (A) CA with normal labyrinth and (B) CA with a dilated vestibule (CADV).

1. CA with normal labyrinth (**Fig. 4.9**):
   In this anomaly there is:
   - Absence of cochlea, and
   - Normally developed vestibule and SCCs.

2. CA with a dilated vestibule (CADV) (**Fig. 4.10**):
   In this anomaly there is:
   - Absence of cochlea, and
   - Dilated vestibule and SCCs.

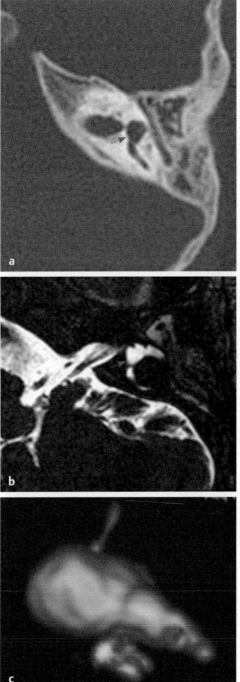

Fig. 4.9 (a) HRCT temporal bone, bone window and **(b)** MRI CISS sequence, axial section shows normal vestibule (pink arrow) and absent cochlea **(c)** 3D reconstructed image showing cochlear aplasia.

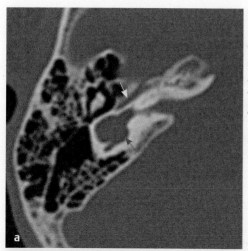

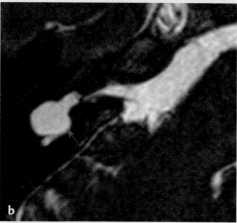

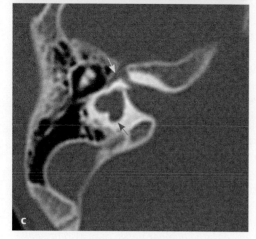

Fig. 4.10 **(a, c)** HRCT temporal bone, bone window and **(b)** MRI CISS sequence, axial section shows dilated vestibule (pink arrow) with anteriorly displaced facial nerve (yellow arrow) and absent cochlea.

Table 4.1 Differences between CADV and CC

Features	CADV	CC
Cochlea	Absent	The cochlear component present anterior to IAC
Vestibule	Dilated and located posterolateral to IAC	The vestibular component present posterior to IAC
IAC	Enters into the anterior-most part of the cavity	Enters into the center of the cavity
Cochlear nerve on 3T MRI (Stenver's projection)	Absent	Cochleovestibular nerve complex present, occasionally cochlear nerve may be seen separately
Behavioral audiometry	Response is absent	Responses present
Cochlear implantation	Contraindicated and ABI is an option for hearing rehabilitation	Option for hearing rehabilitation

Abbreviations: ABI, Auditory brainstem implant; CADV, cochlear aplasia with a dilated vestibule; CC, common cavity; IAC, internal auditory canal, MRI, magnetic resonance imaging.

It is important to differentiate between CADV and CC malformation radiologically prior to CI, as an attempt of CI in CADV patients where there is an absence of cochlea and cochlear nerve may result in no hearing benefit to the patient after surgery. The difference between CADV and CC malformation is enumerated in **Table 4.1**.

Common Cavity

The CC malformation was first described by Edward Cock in 1838. CC occurs as a result of developmental arrest during the fourth and fifth week of gestation[18] when the differentiation of inner ear structures into cochlea and vestibule occurs.

Important features of CC are:

1. It is defined as a single, large, ovoid or round structure, representing cochlea and vestibule (**Fig. 4.11**).
2. This cavity contains neural elements of both cochlea and vestibule.
3. Rudimentary parts of the SCC can be present.
4. The IAC is well developed and enters the midportion (center) of the cavity.
5. In most of the cases, a common cochleovestibular nerve (CVN) is present and occasionally a separate cochlear nerve may also be seen.
6. CI is an effective treatment option for hearing in CC; however, the hearing performance depends on the number of cochlear nerve fibers present in the cochleovestibular bundle which can be evaluated by behavioral audiometry responses.

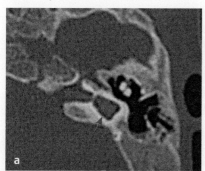

Fig. 4.11 **(a, c)** HRCT temporal bone, bone window and **(b, d)** MRI CISS sequence, axial section shows internal acoustic canal (red star) entering the common cavity (pink arrow) in the center.

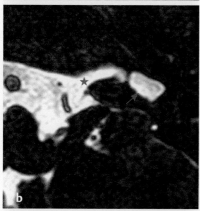

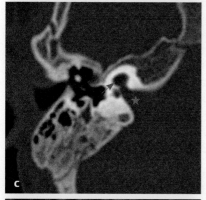

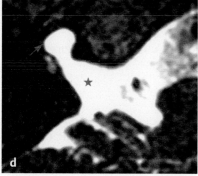

7. The surgical approach for CI is via a transmastoid banana-shaped labyrinthotomy which was first described by McElveen et al.[19]
8. As the neural elements are mainly located at the periphery of the cavity, straight electrodes are preferred. Precurved modiolar hugging and half banded electrodes need to be avoided in such cases.
9. The length of the electrode array required can be calculated prior to surgery by using the formula $2\pi r$, where r is the radius of CC.

A recent study by Nora et al[20] mentions the use of 3D reformation images to differentiate between CADV and CC, as routine HRCT and MRI may underestimate the malformation, especially when the resolution is poor. In this study, a line was drawn along the longitudinal axis of the IAC and another along the medial border of the vestibular part of the inner ear extended along the posterior limit of the IAC as shown in **Fig. 4.12**. The cochlear portion of the cavity was considered present if the CC was located anterior and was said to be absent if the CC was present only posterior to the IAC.

Cochlear Hypoplasias

CH by definition has smaller external dimensions, length as well as height, so the cochlear duct length is less than 25 mm. These are the most interesting malformations because they present in various ways. Hearing may be normal or there may be profound loss; conductive, sensorineural, or mixed hearing loss. Patients with pure conductive hearing loss (specially those with CH3 and CH4) may benefit from stapes surgery. Cochlear nerve deficiency is frequent in CH. As the cochlea is hypoplastic, the promontory is flat and many times the round window is not that well visualized. Facial nerve may also be running an anomalous course. As the turns are smaller and narrower, it is better to use smaller and slimmer electrodes. In his latest modifications to the classification, Sennaroglu has divided CH into four types.

Cochlear Hypoplasia Type 1 (CH1) (Bud-like Cochlea)

Cochlea is visualized like a small bud, arising from the IAC. No modiolus and interscalar septa are identified (**Fig. 4.13**).

Cochlear Hypoplasia Type 2 (CH2)

It is also known as cystic hypoplastic cochlea. Important features of CH2 include (**Fig. 4.14**):

1. Absent modiolus.
2. Absent interscalar septa.
3. Vestibule and VA may be enlarged.
4. There might be a defect between IAC and cochlea, leading to higher chances of cerebrospinal fluid (CSF) gusher during surgery.

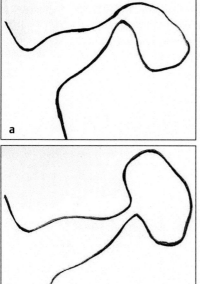

Fig. 4.12 Difference between CADV and CC, **(a)** line diagram of CADV, **(b)** line diagram of CC, **(c)** 3D reconstruction image with cochlear portion present anterior to the longitudinal axis of IAC, and **(d)** 3D reconstruction image with cochlear portion absent anterior to the longitudinal axis of IAC.

5. Stapedial footplate defect may be present leading to CSF otorrhea and recurrent meningitis.
6. As there is no modiolus, the nerve endings are along the periphery of the cochlea. Therefore the best electrodes to be used here would be full banded lateral wall electrodes.
7. In view of chances of CSF gusher, the surgeon should be prepared for dealing with it. Some of the things include: bigger cochleostomy, let the CSF drain out before insertion of electrode array, FORM electrode (proximal part of array having a conical stopper), good sealing of the cochleostomy by tissues, be prepared to use tissue glue and lumbar drain and in worst cases subtotal petrosectomy may be needed.
8. These features are similar to IP1, however the major difference is that cochlea is smaller than 25 mm in CH2.

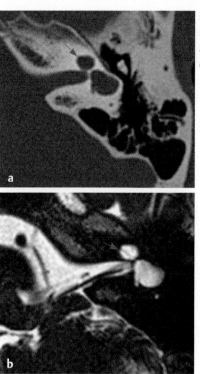

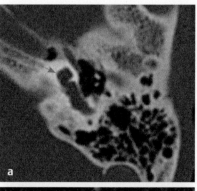

Fig. 4.13 (a) HRCT temporal bone, bone window and **(b)** MRI CISS sequence, axial section shows a small bud-like cochlea (pink arrow) in CH1.

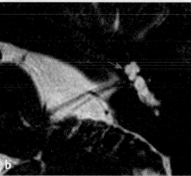

Fig. 4.14 (a) HRCT temporal bone, bone window and **(b)** MRI CISS sequence, axial section shows small cystic cochlea (blue arrow) with normal external outline with absent modiolus and interscalar septa.

Cochlear Hypoplasia Type 3 (CH3)

Its important features include (**Fig. 4.15**):

1. Fewer number of turns.
2. Shorter modiolus.
3. Shorter interscalar septa.
4. It looks like a normal cochlea, but is shorter and with fewer turns.

Cochlear Hypoplasia Type 4 (CH4)

Features of CH4 are (**Fig. 4.16**):

1. Normal basal turn.
2. Middle and apical turns are hypoplastic and located anteriorly.
3. Facial nerve runs an anomalous course.

Incomplete Partitions

These comprise a group of cochlear anomalies where the differentiation between the cochlea and the vestibule is clear cut. The differentiating feature from CHs is that in IP the cochlea is of normal length, that is, more than 25 mm. These are divided into three types on the basis of modiolus and inter scalar septum (**Table 4.2**).

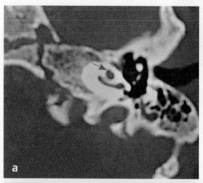
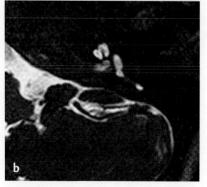

Fig. 4.15 (a) HRCT temporal bone, bone window and pink arrow points towards fewer number of turns of cochlea. **(b)** MRI CISS sequence, axial section shows CH3.

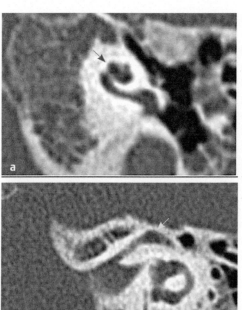

Fig. 4.16   (a, b) HRCT temporal bone, bone window, axial section shows and facial nerve (yellow arrow) is seen running an abnormal course in labyrinthine segment. **(c)** MRI CISS sequence, axial sections show CH4 in which cochlea (pink arrow) has hypoplastic and anteriorly placed middle and apical turns with normal basal turn and an anteriorly placed facial nerve.

Table 4.2   Differences between IP 1, 2, and 3

Deformity	Modiolus	Interscalar septa
IP1	Absent	Absent
IP2	Deficient in apical part	Deficient in apical part
IP3	Absent	Present

Abbreviation: IP, incomplete partitions.

Incomplete Partition Type 1 (IP1)

Important features of IP1 (also known as cystic cochleovestibular malformation) are (**Fig. 4.17**):

1. Normal external architecture.
2. Absent modiolus.
3. Absent interscalar septa.

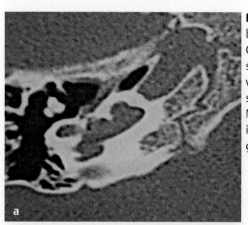

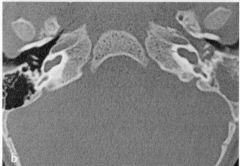

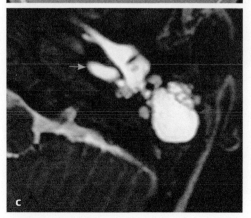

Fig. 4.17 **(a, b)** HRCT temporal bone, bone window and **(c)** MRI CISS sequence, axial sections show IP1. Cochlea (blue arrow) without modiolus and interscalar septum, and bright signal on MRI on left side indicates CSF in middle ear (pink arrow) and going into the eustachian tube.

4. Dilated vestibule.
5. There might be a defect between IAC and cochlea, leading to higher chances (approximately 50%) of CSF gusher during surgery.
6. Stapedial footplate defect may be present leading to CSF otorrhea/otorhinorrhea and recurrent meningitis (**Fig. 4.17**).
7. As there is no modiolus, the nerve endings are along the periphery of the cochlea. Therefore the best electrodes to be used here would be full banded lateral wall electrodes.
8. In view of chances of CSF gusher, the surgeon should be prepared for dealing with it. Some of the things include: bigger cochleostomy, let the CSF drain out before insertion of electrode array, FORM electrode (proximal part of array having a conical stopper), good sealing of the cochleostomy by tissues, be prepared to use tissue glue and lumbar drain and in worst cases subtotal petrosectomy may be needed.

Incomplete Partition Type 2 (IP 2)

Important features of IP2 are (**Fig. 4.18**):

1. Apical part of the modiolus and the corresponding interscalar septa are defective.
2. Apical part of the cochlea looks cystic due to the confluence of middle and apical turns.
3. Modini's deformity: triad of IP2, EVA and dilated vestibule.
4. Hearing may be normal to profound loss (progressive loss).
5. Mild perilymph ooze may be there (no CSF gusher).
6. Any kind of electrode may be used, however complete cochlear coverage should not be an aim.

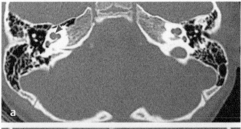
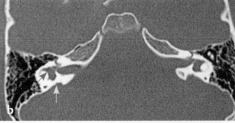

Fig. 4.18 (a, b) HRCT temporal bone, bone window, axial sections show Mondini dysplasia: IP2 - with cystic apical part of cochlea (pink arrow), dilated vestibule (blue arrow), and EVA (yellow arrow).

Incomplete Partition Type 3 (IP3)

Important features of IP3 are (**Fig. 4.19**):

1. Absent modiolus.
2. Interscalar septa present.
3. X-linked deafness.
4. There is a defect between IAC and cochlea, leading to CSF gusher during surgery (100%).
5. As there is no modiolus, the nerve endings are along the periphery of the cochlea. Therefore, the best electrodes to be used here would be full banded lateral wall electrodes.
6. Patients may present with conductive or mixed hearing loss and there have been instances when these patients have been taken up for stapes surgery. If a stapedotomy is done in such patients, intraoperative CSF gusher is encountered which then needs to be repaired and the surgery turns out to be futile. These patients invariably land up with profound SNHL requiring CI.
7. In view of 100% probability of CSF gusher, the surgeon should be prepared for dealing with it. Some of the things include: bigger cochleostomy, let the CSF drain out before insertion of electrode array, FORM electrode (proximal part of array having a conical stopper), good sealing of the cochleostomy by tissues, be prepared to use tissue glue and lumbar drain and in worst cases subtotal petrosectomy may be needed.
8. Also due to big communication between cochlea and IAC, there are chances that electrode array may get misplaced into IAC. Therefore this should be cross-checked intraoperatively with a C-arm. If it

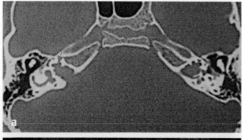
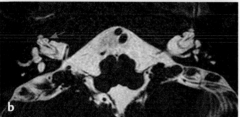

Fig. 4.19 (a) HRCT temporal bone, bone window and **(b)** MRI CISS sequence, axial sections show IP3 (blue arrow) - cochlea has interscalar septum without modiolus and with bilateral dilated internal acoustic canal.

is found to be so, then the electrode array should be removed and inserted again in a different direction, usually antero-superiorly. Electrode array may also be inserted with help of intraoperative fluoroscopy guidance.

9. Facial nerve anomalies may be present.

Sawai Man Singh Classification

Classifications in general, and specifically those relevant to cochleovestibular malformations (CVM), are required for a few basic reasons to make the things easier. The problem with the Sennaroglu et al classification is that overlapping or intermediate forms exist, which creates confusion. This confusion is worsened by the fact that diagnosis of CH is very subjective. There is currently no literature describing how to radiologically measure the length of a malformed cochlea. Thus, there can be overlap between various types of IP and CH. For example, it is sometimes difficult to differentiate between IP type II and CH type III, and IP type I and CH type II. Furthermore, the many additions to the definitions of these terms make it difficult for people to remember and follow this classification. This also leads to problems with uniformity, which is another reason why we need a standard classification. The complex nature of this classification makes it tough for surgeons, audiologists, and speech and language pathologists to understand. Uniformity can be lost even while communicating within the team, which leads to problems in reporting the results.

Another major reason why we need another classification is for treatment planning and predicting complications. Sennaroglu et al's classification[3] can indicate this information, but in a complex manner. For example, if we were to examine various types of CH and IP, and predict which of these have a higher chance of a CSF gusher, then it would be CH type II, and IP types I and III. For any surgeon, a classification that immediately indicates that particular terminology is associated with higher chances of CSF gusher would make more sense and be easier to remember. If not one term, then at least the terms should be in a sequence and not haphazardly placed. Another major reason for a new classification is for predicting prognosis. The terms used in all classifications, be they for angiofibroma or malignancy, or any other disease, usually go from good to bad prognosis, or vice versa. However, this is not seen in this classification. For example, prognosis of IP type II is better than IP types I and III. Furthermore, it is difficult to prognosticate various types of CH and IP. In short, the present classification systems are not adequate for five major reasons. Classification should: make things easier for user, provide uniformity, enable treatment planning (including electrode selection), and allow the prediction of complications and prognosis. Thus, a new, simpler and more clinical classification, with well-delineated types and definitions, is needed.

The SMS classification of CVM[7] took into consideration three features of cochlear anatomy, namely cochlear morphology, the modiolus, and the lamina cribrosa (**Fig. 4.20**).

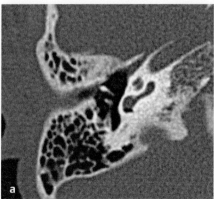

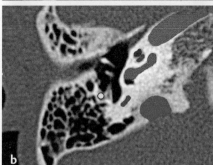

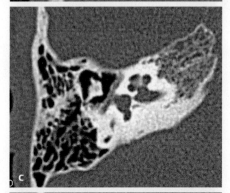

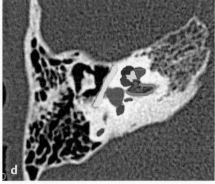

Fig. 4.20 HRCT temporal bone, axial section, bone window show **(a, b, c, d)** (█ light blue) modiolus, (█ purple) apical turn of cochlea, (█ dark pink) middle turn of cochlea, (█ pink) posterior SCC, (yellow) tympanic segment of facial nerve, (█ brown) vestibule and singular canal, (light green) lateral SCC, (█ dark green) IAC, *(Continued)*

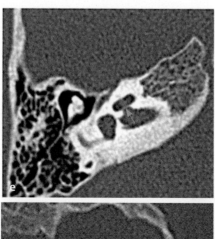

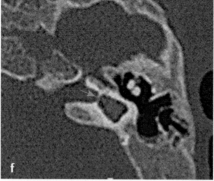

Fig. 4.20 *(Continued)* **(e)** lamina cribrosa (green arrow) in normal cochlea and **(f)** lamina cribrosa (green arrow in abnormal cochlea).

Table 4.3   SMS classification of cochleovestibular malformations

CVM type	Cochlear morphology	Modiolus	Lamina cribrosa	Others
I	Normal	Normal	Normal	Abnormal
IIa	Abnormal	Complete but smaller	Normal	+/–
IIb	Abnormal	Partially defective	Normal	+/–
IIIa	Abnormal	Absent	Normal	+/–
IIIb	Abnormal	Absent	Deficient	+/–
IV	Absent	Absent	Absent	+/–

Abbreviations: CVM, cochleovestibular malformations; SMS, Sawai Man Singh.

Inner ear anomalies other than cochlear anomalies, for example an EVA or vestibular dysplasia, were kept in the "others" category. IAC anomalies or cochlear nerve anomalies were dealt with separately, and were therefore not made a part of this classification. **Table 4.3** outlines the details of this classification.

CVM Type I

Features of CVM type I are (**Fig. 4.21**) as follows:

1. Cochlea is normal.
2. Involves extracochlear parts of the labyrinth like dysplastic vestibule, dysplastic or absent SCCs or EVA.
3. All types of electrodes can be used.
4. Surgery is the same as that for normal cochlea except mild perilymph oozer in EVA.
5. Results are the same as normal cochlea.

CVM Type II

Features of CVM type II are (**Fig. 4.22**) as follows:

1. Cochlear morphology is not normal.
2. Modiolus is present, however in type IIa the modiolus is complete but smaller and in type IIb it is partially defective in the upper half.
3. The lamina cribrosa is normal so there is no communication between IAC and cochlea.
4. All electrodes can be used.
5. Surgery is the same as that for normal cochlea except mild perilymph oozer in few patients.
6. Results are the same as normal cochlea.

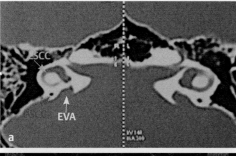
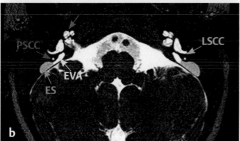

Fig. 4.21 **(a)** HRCT temporal bone, bone window and **(b)** MRI CISS sequence, axial sections show SMS CVM type 1 with normal cochlea and EVA (yellow arrow), PSCC (pink arrow), LSCC (blue arrow), and endolymphatic sac (ES, green arrow).

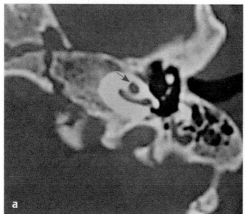

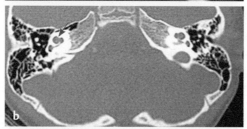

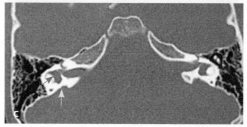

Fig. 4.22 HRCT temporal bone, bone window, axial sections show CVM type II with **(a)** type IIa and **(b, c)** type 2b with Mondini dysplasia with cystic apical part of cochlea (pink arrow), dilated vestibule (blue arrow) and EVA (yellow arrow).

CVM Type III

Features of CVM type III are (**Fig. 4.23**) as follows:

1. Cochlear morphology is not normal.
2. Modiolus is absent.
3. Lamina cribrosa is normal in type IIIa and deficient or absent in type IIIb leading to big communication between IAC and cochlea in latter.
4. As there is no modiolus, the nerve endings are along the periphery of the cochlea. Therefore the best electrodes to be used here would be full banded lateral wall electrodes.
5. Chances of CSF gusher are high in type IIIb, therefore the surgeon should be prepared for dealing with it. Some of the things include: bigger cochleostomy, let the CSF drain out before insertion of electrode array, FORM electrode (proximal part of array having a conical stopper), good sealing of the cochleostomy by tissues, be

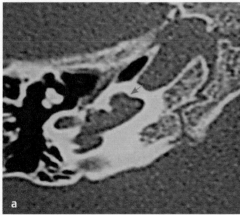

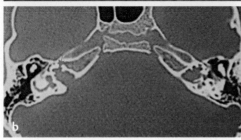

Fig. 4.23 HRCT temporal bone, bone window, axial sections show CVM type III (blue arrow) with **(a)** type IIIa (absent modiolus, lamina cribrosa present) and **(b)** type IIIb (absent modiolus and absent lamina cribrosa).

   prepared to use tissue glue and lumbar drain and in worst cases subtotal petrosectomy may be needed.

6. Also in type IIIb, due to big communication between cochlea and IAC, there are chances that electrode array may get misplaced into IAC. Therefore, this should be cross-checked intraoperatively with a C-arm. If it is found to be so, then the electrode array should be removed and inserted again in different direction, usually antero-superiorly. Electrode array may also be inserted with help of intraoperative fluoroscopy guidance.

CVM Type IV

Features of CVM type IV are (**Fig. 4.24**) as follows:

1. Cochlea is absent.
2. Vestibular components may or may not be normally developed.
3. CI is contraindicated and the patient needs an auditory brainstem implant.

The authors find this classification simple and practical, covering all malformation types. This means it can be used universally without any confusion. It can also be utilized to predict outcomes without any overlap of terminologies.

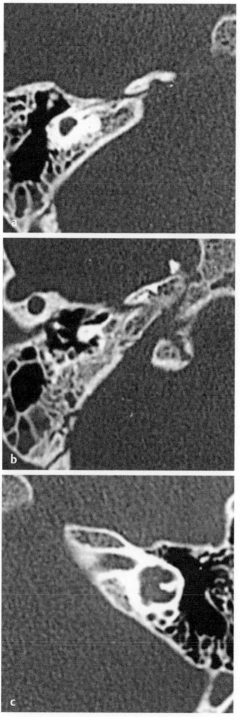

Fig. 4.24 HRCT temporal bone, bone window, axial sections show CVM type IV, **(a)** rudimentary otocyst without IAC, **(b)** CLA, and **(c)** cochlear aplasia.

Cochlear Aperture Anomalies

1. The cochlear aperture is also known as cochlear fossette, or bony cochlear nerve canal (BCNC), that connects the cochlea to the IAC and transmits the cochlear nerve from the cochlea to the IAC (**Fig. 4.25**).
2. Cochlear aperture is clearly visualized in the mid modiolar view and is measured in axial sections of the HRCT temporal bone (**Fig. 4.25**).
3. Cochlear aperture can be normal, hypoplastic, aplastic, or wide.
4. Cochlear aperture aplasia and hypoplasia are most commonly seen with CHARGE association.
5. Cochlear aperture is considered hypoplastic (**Fig. 4.26**) if the width of the BCNC is less than 1.4 mm.[21]
6. Cochlear aperture is considered to be aplastic (**Fig. 4.27**) when the BCNC is completely replaced by bone or there is no canal seen.
7. Cochlear aperture is said to be wide when the width of the BCNC is more than 3 mm. This anomaly is most commonly seen in X-linked progressive hearing loss (SMS CVM type IIIb), wherein the bony partition between the IAC and the cochlea is absent. CI in such cases may be complicated by CSF gusher intraoperatively.
8. Cochlear aperture abnormalities may be accompanied by a narrow or a dilated IAC in most of the cases.

Cochlear Nerve Anomalies

The classification of CVN is of vital importance in the management of inner ear malformations. In MRI CISS/FIESTA sequence, oblique sagittal sections, typically four separate nerves, that is, facial nerve anterosuperior, cochlear nerve (CN) anteroinferior, superior vestibular nerve posterosuperior, and inferior vestibular nerve posteroinferior are clearly distinguished at the fundus of IAC. Casselman et al described cochlear nerve hypoplasia or aplasia based on its dimensions in relation to the ipsilateral facial nerve.[22] Studies mention that the CN is of similar size or larger than the facial nerve in 64% of cases and the relative size of the four nerves is symmetrical with the contralateral IAC in 70% of cases.[23] The CN size is correlated with spiral ganglion cell population, and thus may help predict the outcome of cochlear implantation.

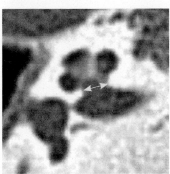

Fig. 4.25 HRCT temporal bone, axial view, bone window shows the measurement of the cochlear aperture (BCNC) at mid-modiolar level.

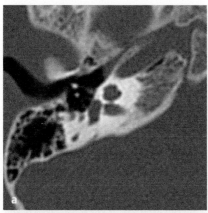

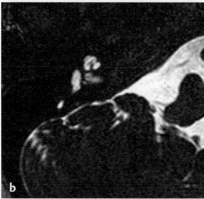

Fig. 4.26 **(a)** HRCT temporal bone window and **(b)** MRI CISS sequence, axial sections shows narrow cochlear aperture with hypoplastic cochlear nerve.

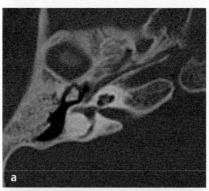

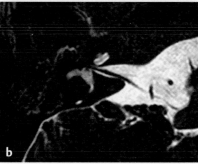

Fig. 4.27 **(a)** HRCT temporal bone window and **(b)** MRI CISS sequence, axial sections shows complete cochlear aperture stenosis with cochlear nerve aplasia.

Casselman et al[24] came up with a classification in which they divided the CVN anomalies into following types:

- Type I: No CVN seen. Only facial nerve present.
- Type IIa: Absence of CN with dysplastic labyrinth.
- Type IIb: Absence of CN with normal labyrinth.
- Type III: Isolated aplasia of vestibular nerve (never reported till now).

The newer classification by Sennaroglu divides CVN abnormalities into six types.

Normal Cochlear Nerve

1. On oblique sagittal sections, a separate CN is seen in the anteroinferior part of the IAC.
2. The size of CN is similar when compared to the contralateral normal side (**Fig. 4.28**).
3. The size of the CN is similar or slightly larger than the ipsilateral facial nerve sections where we see the CN entering the modiolus of the cochlea (**Fig. 4.28**).

Hypoplastic Cochlear Nerve

1. Separate CN is seen anteroinferiorly.
2. The size of the CN is smaller when compared to the contralateral normal side (**Fig. 4.29**).
3. The size of the CN is smaller than the ipsilateral facial nerve.
4. Most commonly seen in cases with BCNC stenosis or atresia, narrow IAC, and anomalies like CH.

Absent Cochlear Nerve

1. No nerve is seen in the anteroinferior part of the IAC, on MRI oblique sagittal sections (**Fig. 4.30**).
2. Most commonly seen in malformations such as CA, but can occasionally be seen in CH.

Normal Cochleovestibular Nerve

1. A single CVN complex originates at the brainstem and then separates into CN and SVN and inferior vestibular nerves in the IAC (**Fig. 4.31**).
2. In malformations such as a CC, CVN enters the cavity without separating into individual nerves.
3. If the CVN is of size 1.5 to 2 times larger than the ipsilateral facial nerve or similar in size when compared to the contralateral CVN, the CVN is considered normal.

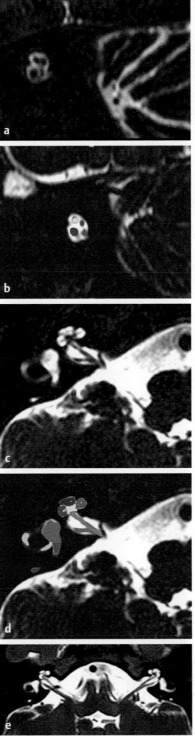

Fig. 4.28 MRI CISS/FIESTA sequence, **(a, b)** oblique sagittal images at fundus of internal acoustic canal and **(c, d, e)** axial sections show normal cochlear nerve larger than facial nerve. (■ Yellow, facial nerve; ■ brown, superior vestibular nerve above and inferior vestibular nerve below; ■ blue, cochlear nerve; ■ Pink - posterior SCC, ■ Purple - apical turn of cochlea, ■ Dark Pink - middle turn of cochlea, ■ Light pink- basal turn of cochlea, ■ Light green - lateral SCC, ■ Light blue - modiolus, and ■ Red arrow shows Rosenthal's canal (RC)).

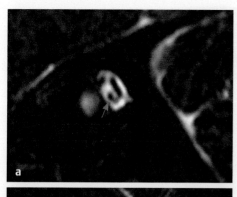

Fig. 4.29 MRI CISS/FIESTA sequence, **(a)** oblique sagittal images at fundus of internal acoustic canal and **(b)** axial sections show hypoplastic cochlear nerve (blue arrow) smaller than the facial nerve.

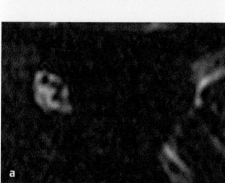

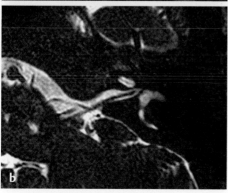

Fig. 4.30 MRI CISS/FIESTA sequence, **(a)** oblique sagittal images at fundus of internal acoustic canal and **(b)** axial sections show absent cochlear nerve.

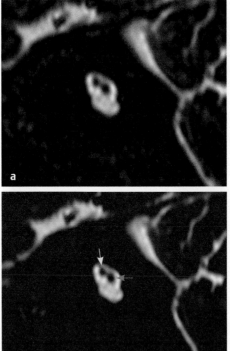

Fig. 4.31 **(a)** MRI CISS/FIESTA sequence, oblique sagittal images at fundus of internal acoustic canal and **(b)** show vestibulocochlear nerve (brown arrow) and facial nerve (yellow arrow).

Hypoplastic CVN

1. When CVN is smaller than the contralateral CVN or ipsilateral facial nerve (**Fig. 4.32**).
2. Commonly seen in CC malformations.

Absent CVN

1. CVN is absent (**Fig. 4.33**).
2. Seen in Michel deformity.
3. Only a single nerve, that is, facial nerve can be seen in Michel deformity with absent IAC.

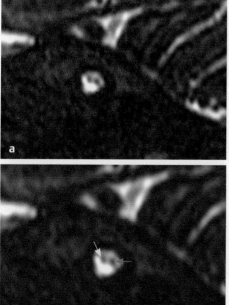

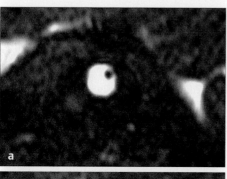

Fig. 4.32 **(a)** MRI CISS/FIESTA sequence, oblique sagittal reformation images at fundus of internal acoustic canal and **(b)** show vestibulocochlear nerve (brown arrow) smaller than facial nerve (yellow arrow).

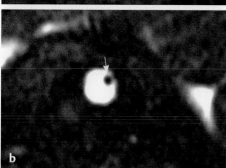

Fig. 4.33 **(a)** MRI CISS/FIESTA sequence, oblique sagittal images at fundus of IAC and **(b)** show single facial nerve (yellow arrow).

Internal Acoustic Canal Anomalies

The IAC is a smooth, cylindrical canal that extends from the porus acusticus at the cerebellopontine angle medially to the fundus laterally, adjacent to the inner ear. The IAC transmits the branches of the vestibulocochlear nerves, that is, cochlear nerve, superior and inferior vestibular nerve, singular nerve, and the intracanalicular segment of the facial nerve. Several studies have shown a strong correlation between the width of the IAC and associated CVN anomalies. The normal IAC width is 2 to 8 mm.[25,26]

The width of the IAC is measured in axial sections of the HRCT temporal bone by drawing a line perpendicular to the long axis of IAC at its mid point (**Fig. 4.34a**). The height and length of the IAC are measured on coronal sections. Height is measured by drawing a line through the mid canal (**Fig. 4.34b**). The upper limit for the height of the IAC is around 8 mm and for the length is generally 10 mm. The normal orientation angle of IAC is 60 to 65°. It is measured by drawing a line anteriorly from an axis drawn along the posterior petrous edge intersecting with a line drawn along the posterior wall of the IAC (**Fig. 4.34c**).[26]

IAC anomalies are classified into three categories based on the width, length, and duplication. IAC can be narrow or widened based on its width. It could be foreshortened, tortuous, and bulbous based on the height or posteriorly angulated.

Narrow Internal Acoustic Canal

IAC is said to be narrow or stenotic if the width is less than 2 mm (**Figs. 4.35** and **4.36**).[9,27] Most of the cases IAC stenosis may be accompanied by BCNC stenosis. Several studies have shown the presence of a hypoplastic or aplastic CN associated with a narrow IAC intraoperatively.

Widened Internal Acoustic Canal

IAC is considered to be wide if the width is more than 8 mm. It can be bulbous or fusiform (**Figs. 4.37** and **4.38**). Several syndromes such as CHARGE, Goldenhar, Apert, Patau are frequently associated with widened IAC.[28] Bulbous and widened IAC is a classical feature of X-linked mixed hearing loss, in which there is incomplete separation or absence of lamina cribrosa between the IAC and the basal turn of the cochlea, thus increasing the risk of CSF gusher (as in SMS CVM type IIIb).

Duplicated Internal Acoustic Canal

It is a very rare congenital anomaly and very few cases have been reported in literature. In this, there is a bony septum that divides IAC into anterosuperior and posteroinferior parts. The anterosuperior portion is usually bigger in size (**Fig. 4.39**).

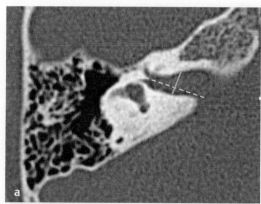

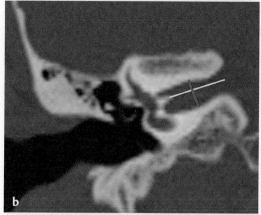

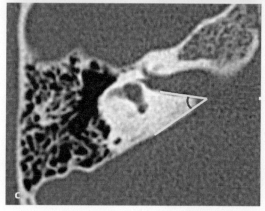

Fig. 4.34 HRCT temporal bone, bone window, **(a)** axial section shows measurement of the width of the internal acoustic canal (IAC) at its midpoint (yellow dotted line, long axis of IAC), **(b)** coronal section showing the measurement of the height of IAC, **(c)** axial section shows measurement of the angle of orientation of IAC.

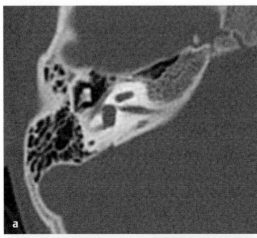

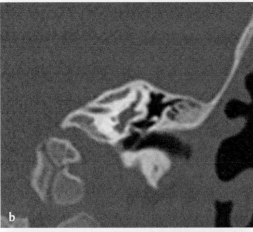

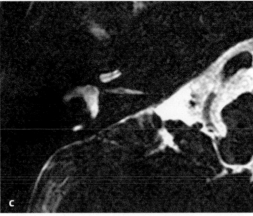

Fig. 4.35 HRCT temporal bone, bone window, **(a)** axial section, **(b)** coronal section, and **(c)** MRI CISS sequence axial section shows narrow internal acoustic canal in normal inner ear.

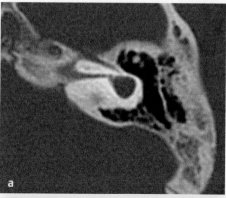

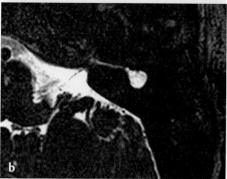

Fig. 4.36 (a) HRCT temporal bone, bone window and **(b)** MRI CISS sequence axial section shows narrow internal acoustic canal in anomalous inner ear.

Summary of Cochlear Malformations

In order to make these malformations simpler and more practical, authors are trying to describe them by means of some hypothetical diagrams.

Fig. 4.40 explains about normal cochlear anatomy, the important structures like the turns, modiolus, interscalar septa, and lamina cribrosa.

Fig. 4.41 talks about the scenario when the cochlea is normal but the rest of the inner ear can be affected (e.g., dysplastic vestibule/SCC/EVA). As the electrode goes only till the initial part of the middle turn, the results do not change and any type of electrode array (full banded/half banded; lateral wall/perimodiolar/midscalar) can be used.

Fig. 4.42 shows the scenario when the modiolus is shorter in size or it is defective in the upper half. As the electrode goes only till the initial part of the middle turn, the results do not change and any type of electrode array (full banded/half banded; lateral wall/perimodiolar/midscalar) can be used. This includes IP2 and CH3 (SMS CVM type 2).

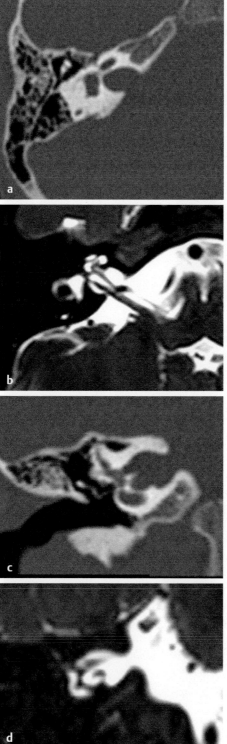

Fig. 4.37 **(a, c)** HRCT temporal bone, bone window, **(a)** Axial and **(c)** coronal sections and **(b, d)** MRI CISS sequence, **(b)** axial sections and **(d)** coronal sections show widened internal acoustic canal with normal inner ear.

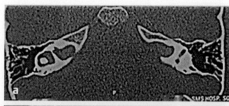

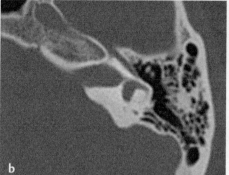

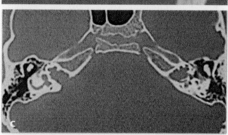

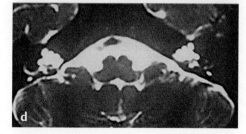

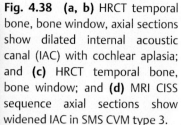

Fig. 4.38 **(a, b)** HRCT temporal bone, bone window, axial sections show dilated internal acoustic canal (IAC) with cochlear aplasia; and **(c)** HRCT temporal bone, bone window; and **(d)** MRI CISS sequence axial sections show widened IAC in SMS CVM type 3.

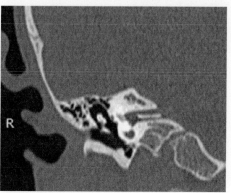

Fig. 4.39 HRCT temporal bone, coronal sections, bone window shows duplicated internal acoustic canal.

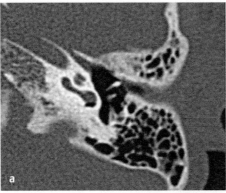

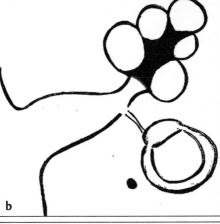

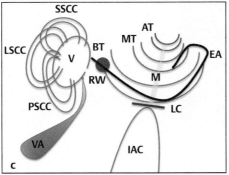

Fig. 4.40 **(a)** normal radiological anatomy of cochlea, **(b)** line diagram of normal cochlea, **(c)** schematic representation of electrode insertion in normal cochlea (going only up to initial part of middle turn) (AT, apical turn; IAC, internal acoustic canal; MT, middle turn; BT, basal turn; M, modiolus; RW, round window; SSCC, superior semicircular canal; LSCC, lateral semicircular canal; PSCC, posterior semicircular canal; EA, electrode array; LC, lamina cribrosa; V,vetibule).

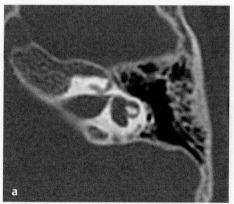

Fig. 4.41 **(a)** Normal radiological anatomy of cochlea with dilated vestibule, **(b)** line diagram of normal cochlea with dilated vestibule and EVA, **(c)** schematic representation of electrode insertion in normal cochlea with dilated vestibule and EVA.

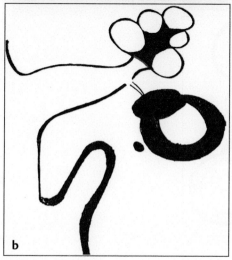

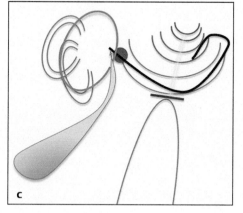

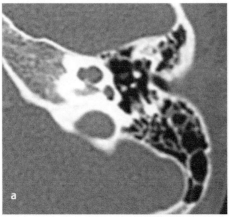

Fig. 4.42 (a) Abnormal radiological anatomy of cochlea with fused apical and middle turns, **(b)** line diagram of abnormal cochlea with fused middle and apical turns with a defective modiolus, **(c)** schematic representation of electrode insertion in abnormal cochlea with defective modiolus in the upper half and **(d)** schematic representation of electrode insertion in abnormal cochlea with shorter modiolus.

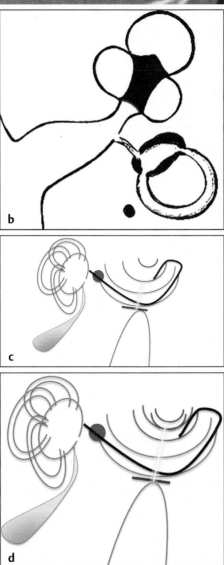

Fig. 4.43 tries to explain the scenario when the modiolus is absent but interscalar septa are intact and lamina cribrosa is absent (IP3 SMS CVM type IIIb). As the modiolus is absent, the nerve endings are present along the periphery of cochlea and therefore half banded/modiolus hugging electrodes should not be used. These electrodes will be facing away from the nerve endings and the precurved electrode array may coil on its own (**Fig. 4.43d**). Full banded lateral wall electrode arrays are best suited for such an anomaly (**Fig. 4.43e**).

Fig. 4.44 shows the scenario when the modiolus and interscalar septa are absent but lamina cribrosa is present (IP1, SMS CVM type IIIa). Just like the last scenario, as the modiolus is absent, the nerve endings are present along the periphery of cochlea and therefore half banded/modiolus hugging electrodes should not be used. These electrodes will be facing away from the nerve endings and the precurved electrode array may coil on its own (**Fig. 4.44d**). Full banded lateral wall electrode arrays are best suited for such an anomaly (**Fig. 4.44e**).

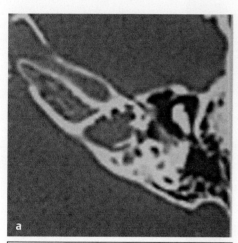

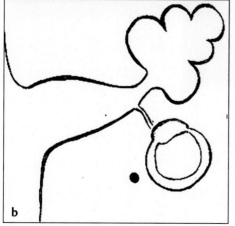

Fig. 4.43 Scenario with abnormal radiological anatomy of cochlea with absent modiolus, absent lamina cribrosa and present interscalar septa, **(a)** abnormal radiological anatomy, **(b)** line diagram. *(Continued)*

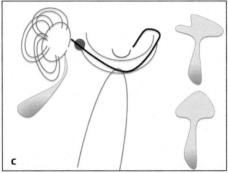

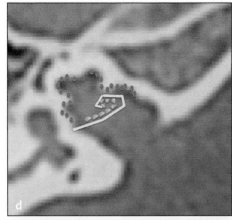

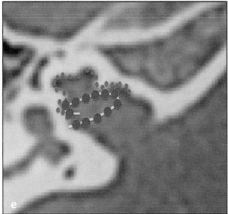

Fig. 4.43 *(Continued)* **(c)** schematic representation of electrode insertion, **(d)** schematic representation of half banded electrode array (yellow) insertion. Half banded electrode arrays are to be avoided in such cases as electrodes (light blue) are facing away from the nerve endings (pink) and the modulus hugging electrode arrays get coiled upon themselves and **(e)** schematic representation of full banded electrode (yellow) insertion, with electrodes (dark blue) seen in close proximity to neural elements (pink) in the periphery.

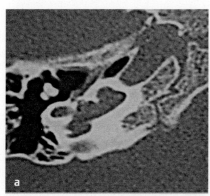

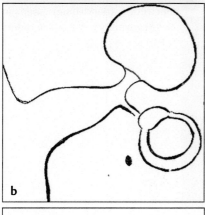

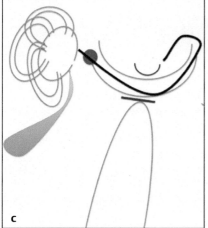

Fig. 4.44 Scenario with abnormal radiological anatomy of cochlea with absent modiolus, lamina cribrosa present and absent interscalar septa, **(a)** abnormal radiological anatomy, **(b)** line diagram, **(c)** schematic representation of electrode insertion. *(Continued)*

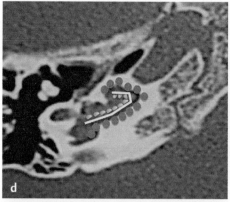

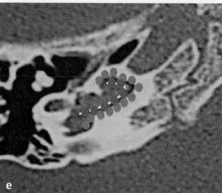

Fig. 4.44 *(Continued)* **(d)** schematic representation of half banded electrode array (yellow) insertion. Half banded electrode arrays are to be avoided in such cases as electrodes (light blue) are facing away from the nerve endings (pink) and the modulus hugging electrode arrays get coiled upon themselves and **(e)** schematic representation of full banded electrode (yellow) insertion, with electrodes (dark blue) seen in close proximity to neural elements (pink) in the periphery.

References

1. Jackler RK, Luxford WM, House WF. Congenital malformations of the inner ear: a classification based on embryogenesis. Laryngoscope 1987; 97(3 Pt 2, Suppl 40)2–14
2. Papsin BC. Cochlear implantation in children with anomalous cochleovestibular anatomy. Laryngoscope 2005; 115(1 Pt 2, Suppl 106)1–26
3. Sennaroğlu L, Bajin MD. Classification and Current Management of Inner Ear Malformations. Balkan Med J 2017;34(5):397–411
4. Mondini C. Anatomica surdi nati sectio; De Bononiensi scientarum et artium institute atque academia commentarii. Bononiae. 1971;7:419–431
5. Phelps PD. Cochlear implants for congenital deformities. J Laryngol Otol 1992;106(11):967–970
6. Sennaroglu L, Saatci I. A new classification for cochleovestibular malformations. Laryngoscope 2002;112(12):2230–2241
7. Grover M, Sharma S, Preetam C, et al. New SMS classification of cochleovestibular malformation and its impact on decision-making. J Laryngol Otol 2019;133(5):368–375
8. Sennaroglu L. Histopathology of inner ear malformations: do we have enough evidence to explain pathophysiology? Cochlear Implants Int 2016;17(1):3–20
9. Sennaroglu L. Cochlear implantation in inner ear malformations—a review article. Cochlear Implants Int 2010;11(1):4–41

10. Monsanto RDC, Sennaroğlu L, Uchiyama M, Sancak IG, Paparella MM, Cureoglu S. Histopathology of inner ear malformations: potential pitfalls for cochlear implantation. Otol Neurotol 2019;40(8):e839–e846

11. Sennaroğlu L, Bajin MD. Incomplete partition type III: a rare and difficult cochlear implant surgical indication. Auris Nasus Larynx 2018;45(1):26–32

12. Valvassori GE, Clemis JD. The large vestibular aqueduct syndrome. Laryngoscope 1978;88(5):723–728

13. Boston M, Halsted M, Meinzen-Derr J, et al. The large vestibular aqueduct: a new definition based on audiologic and computed tomography correlation. Otolaryngol Head Neck Surg 2007;136(6):972–977

14. Wilson DF, Hodgson RS, Talbot JM. Endolymphatic sac obliteration for large vestibular aqueduct syndrome. Am J Otol 1997;18(1):101–106, discussion 106–107

15. Lo WW, Daniels DL, Chakeres DW, et al. The endolymphatic duct and sac. AJNR Am J Neuroradiol 1997;18(5):881–887

16. Sennaroğlu L. Another evidence for pressure transfer mechanism in incomplete partition two anomaly via enlarged vestibular aqueduct. Cochlear Implants Int 2018;19(6):355–357

17. Grover M. Enlarged vestibular aqueduct and cochlear anomalies: just an association or a causal relationship? Cochlear Implants Int 2019;0(0):1–1

18. Cock E. A Contribution to the Pathology of Congenital Deafness. Samuel Highley; 1838

19. McElveen JT Jr, Carrasco VN, Miyamoto RT, Linthicum FH Jr. Cochlear implantation in common cavity malformations using a transmastoid labyrinthotomy approach. Laryngoscope 1997;107(8):1032–1036

20. Weiss NM, Langner S, Mlynski R, Roland P, Dhanasingh A. Evaluating common cavity cochlear deformities using CT images and 3D reconstruction. Laryngoscope 2021;131(2):386–391.

21. Stjernholm C, Muren C. Dimensions of the cochlear nerve canal: a radioanatomic investigation. Acta Otolaryngol 2002;122(1):43–48

22. Casselman JW, Offeciers FE, Govaerts PJ, et al. Aplasia and hypoplasia of the vestibulocochlear nerve: diagnosis with MR imaging. Radiology 1997;202(3):773–781

23. Kim HS, Kim DI, Chung IH, Lee WS, Kim KY. Topographical relationship of the facial and vestibulocochlear nerves in the subarachnoid space and internal auditory canal. AJNR Am J Neuroradiol 1998;19(6):1155–1161

24. Govaerts PJ, Casselman J, Daemers K, De Beukelaer C, Yperman M, De Ceulaer G. Cochlear implants in aplasia and hypoplasia of the cochleovestibular nerve. Otol Neurotol 2003;24(6):887–891

25. Marques SR, Ajzen S, D Ippolito G, Alonso L, Isotani S, Lederman H. Morphometric analysis of the internal auditory canal by computed tomography imaging. Iran J Radiol 2012;9(2):71–78

26. Chetcuti K, Kumbla S. The internal acoustic canal—another review area in paediatric sensorineural hearing loss. Pediatr Radiol 2016;46(4):562–569

27. Masuda S, Usui S, Matsunaga T. High prevalence of inner-ear and/or internal auditory canal malformations in children with unilateral sensorineural hearing loss. Int J Pediatr Otorhinolaryngol 2013;77(2):228–232

28. Bisdas S, Lenarz M, Lenarz T, Becker H. The abnormally dilated internal auditory canal: a non-specific finding or a distinctive pathologic entity. J Neuroradiol 2006;33(4):275–277

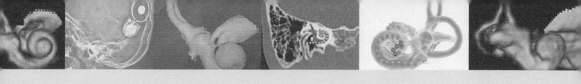

Chapter 5

Inner Ear and Central Pathologies Pertaining to Cochlear Implants

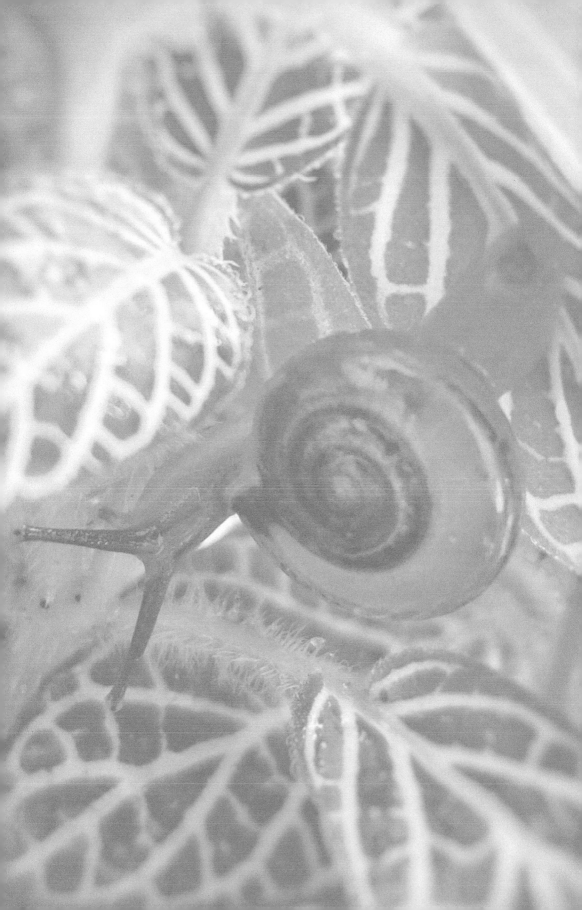

5 Inner Ear and Central Pathologies Pertaining to Cochlear Implants

Introduction

As we read in the last chapter, the surgery and results of cochlear implant (CI) are affected to a great extent by inner ear malformations. They also depend on other inner ear and central pathologies. Many times because of these pathologies, the surgery needs to be done early. At other times, the surgery needs to be delayed till the treatment of the pathology is done. Sometimes, the surgery is contraindicated. All these pathologies do affect the prognosis as well. In this chapter, we will be discussing few of such pathologies.

Labyrinthitis Ossificans

Other than malformations of the inner ear, this is the next most common pathology affecting the inner ear. Labyrinthitis ossificans (LO) is defined as pathological ossification of the membranous labyrinth within the otic capsule in response to an inflammatory or destructive process. LO is usually a sequela of previous infection and can develop through various ways of infection dissemination, such as hematogenic (via cochlear vasculature secondary to viral infections), meningogenic (via cochlear aqueduct from the subarachnoid space), tympanogenic (as a sequela of otitis media, i.e., the spread of infection via the round window),[1] or posttraumatic. The human osseous labyrinth is composed of three layers, that is, endosteal, endochondral, and periosteal layers. LO alters the architecture of the endochondral bone; however, it does not cross the endosteal layer. The lumen of the otic capsule remains patent in the absence of any pathological conditions. In cases of pathological conditions such as meningitis, otosclerosis, Paget's disease, trauma, ototoxicity, malignant infiltration, vascular obliteration of labyrinthine artery, or other infections,[2] the new disorganized woven bone replaces the normal healthy bone and obliterates the spaces of the otic capsule.

Bacterial meningitis is the most common cause of LO. The most common organisms causing meningitis are *Haemophilus influenzae*, *Streptococcus pneumoniae*, and *Neisseria meningitidis*. *Streptococcus pneumoniae* is the most common organism causing deafness post meningitis, which occurs due to the robust inflammatory response to the teichoic acid content in the bacterial cell wall. This tells us the importance of proper immunization at least 2 weeks prior to CI. Several studies report that the pathophysiology of deafness after meningitis is due to the spread of infection from the meninges of the posterior cranial fossa via the cochlear aqueduct to the scala tympani of the basal turn of the cochlea. The most common region to be involved is the scala tympani of the basal turn of the cochlea close to the round window. In these cases, there is an increased concentration of the inflammatory mediators in the region where the cochlear aqueduct drains into the scala tympani explaining the predominant degree of damage in this area. Another reason for increased ossification in the scala tympani of the basal turn is due to reduced perfusion due to the relative decreased blood supply in this region. Ceftazidime is a first-line medical management for the prevention of otogenic and meningogenic labyrinthitis as it reaches higher concentrations in the perilymph and cerebrospinal fluid (CSF). Studies have shown that steroids (dexamethasone) have been shown to reduce the progression of hearing loss in cases of meningitis with *H. influenzae* by inhibiting the synthesis of connective tissues and reducing granulation tissue formation, thus decreasing total collagen formation.

Based on the pathophysiology, Paparella and Sugiura divided LO into three stages:[3]

- Acute stage: In the acute stage, bacteria and leukocytes get accumulated in the perilymphatic spaces but spare the endolymphatic space.
- Fibrous stage: With an ongoing process, there is increased angiogenesis, with fibroblastic proliferation and osteoid deposition (undifferentiated mesenchymal cells) in the perilymphatic spaces.
- Ossification stage: In this stage, both perilymphatic and endolymphatic spaces are obliterated with unorganized woven bone.

LO causes progressive ossification of the cochlea and leads to progressive sensorineural hearing loss of varying degrees. Early imaging, proper audiological follow-up, and early intervention is required in such cases. The best and the only possible chance of hearing rehabilitation is the insertion of a CI electrode early. If LO is bilateral, bilateral CI should be considered as early as possible as the advancing ossification process within the cochlea can preclude a later CI.[4,5,6]

Imaging diagnosis of LO can be made by high-resolution computed tomography (HRCT) scans or magnetic resonance imaging (MRI) of the temporal bones with good resolution and accuracy[7] and it helps to evaluate the possibility of CI.[8] HRCT scans have high sensitivity to identify the late ossified stages of LO, however, it may flounder in detecting early acute and fibrous stages of LO. This is avoided by MRI scans which can identify perilymphatic space fibrosis prior to ossification.

In the chapter on inner ear radiology, we have read about the CT and MRI findings of a normal cochlea. Usually, it is well visualized on T2-weighted (T2W) images in which we get a bright signal because of fluid (**Figs. 5.1** and **5.2b**). Abnormalities on post-meningitis T2W images will appear later than on the contrast-enhanced T1-weighted (T1W) images. The latter will show enhancement in the acute phase (**Fig. 5.2d**). T2W images will show

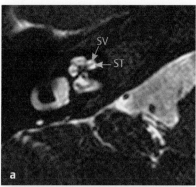

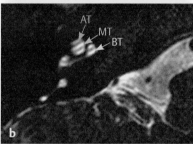

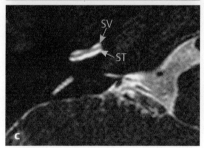

Fig. 5.1 MRI brain T2W CISS/FIESTA sequence, axial sections showing bright fluid signal in: **(a)** ST (green arrow) scala tympani and SV (blue arrow) scala vestibuli of the cochlea. **(b)** Three turns of the cochlea, BT (yellow arrow) basal turn, MT (green arrow) middle turn, and AT (blue arrow) apical turn. **(c)** ST and SV of the basal turn of the cochlea.

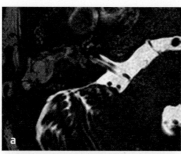

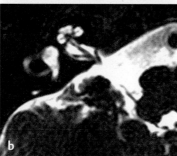

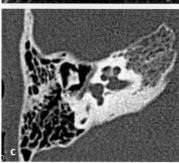

Fig. 5.2 Different stages of labyrinthitis ossificans (LO), MRI CISS/FIESTA sequence, and HRCT temporal bone, bone window, axial sections show: **(a, b, c)** Normal scans showing no enhancement in T1W with contrast, bright fluid signal in T2W and normal HRCT. *(Continued)*

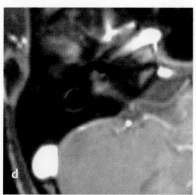

Fig. 5.2 *(Continued)* **(d, e, f)** Acute stage of LO showing enhancement in T1W with contrast **(d)**, bright fluid signal in T2W **(e)**, and normal HRCT **(f)**. *(Continued)*

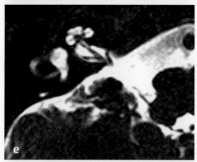

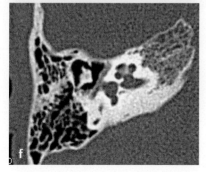

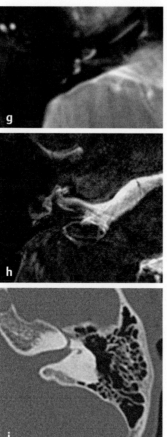

Fig. 5.2 *(Continued)* **(g, h, i)** Fibrosis stage of LO showing mild enhancement in T1W with contrast **(g)**, loss of bright fluid signal in T2W **(h)**, and opacification on HRCT **(i)**. *(Continued)*

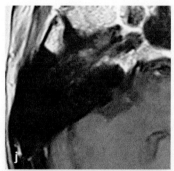

Fig. 5.2 *(Continued)* **(j, k, l)** Ossified stage of LO showing no enhancement in T1W with contrast **(j)**, loss of bright fluid signal in T2W **(k)**, and ossification on HRCT **(l)**. *(Continued)*

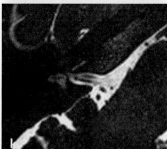

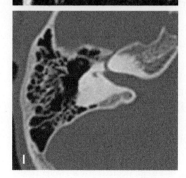

loss of bright (fluid) signal due to either fibrosis (**Fig. 5.2h**) or calcified (**Fig. 5.2k**) tissue. HRCT images are the last to show changes of LO as fibrosis and acute inflammation are not visualized on CT (**Fig. 5.2**). So, if there is any history suggestive of a pathology that may lead to LO, then the surgeon should be careful on reading radiology as it may appear completely normal on CT even though the patient is having early changes of LO. The authors have experienced that only if one cochlea is enhanced on contrast T1W images, it is likely that the normal hearing of the unenhanced cochlea will be preserved. Loss of fluid signal in the lateral semicircular canal should be taken as an early sign of LO, indicating the chance of progression of disease.[9] Various classifications have been put forward based on the opacification seen on the HRCT temporal bone. The initial classification by Balkany and Dreisbach[10] is outlined below.

Cochlear Patency—Balkany and Dreisbach

- C 0: Normal cochlea.
- C 1: Indistinctness of endosteum of the basal turn.
- C 2: Definite narrowing of the basal turn.
- C 3: Bony obliteration of at least a portion of the basal/middle turn or the entire cochlea.

Based on the degree of ossification and surgical approach, Balkany et al classified LO into four stages (**Table 5.1**).[11]

Factors that influence the success of CI include the number of residual spiral ganglion cells, partial versus complete electrode insertion, and duration of deafness before implantation. The loss of spiral ganglion cells is correlated with the degree of fibrosis and ossification. Tremendous advances and newer surgical techniques with the development of specific electrodes have enabled a wider candidacy for CI in cases of LO. Insertion of more electrodes gives a better outcome. Several techniques have been developed to obtain the largest possible number of electrodes implanted in a totally ossified cochlea[5,6,12,13,14,15] and specifically designed CI devices with compressed[16] or double/split arrays.[17]

Table 5.1   Stages of labyrinthitis ossificans as per Balkany et al classification

Stage	Site of ossification	Surgical approach
I (**Fig. 5.3**)	Round window	Cochleostomy
II (**Fig. 5.4**)	Inferior basal turn	Drill: through round window niche
III	Basal turn >180 degrees	
IIIa (**Fig. 5.5**)	180–360 degrees	• Scala vestibuli insertion • Partial drill out with compressed or split electrode array insertion
IIIb (**Fig. 5.6**)	>360 degrees	Total drill out with canal wall up or canal wall down/auditory brainstem implant (ABI)

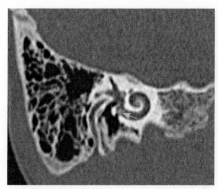

Fig. 5.3 HRCT temporal bone, bone window, oblique sagittal reconstruction images showing LO stage I with ossification (green arrow) confined to the round window region.

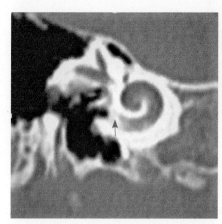

Fig. 5.4 HRCT temporal bone, bone window, oblique sagittal reconstruction image showing LO stage II with ossification (red arrow) in the inferior segment of basal turn.

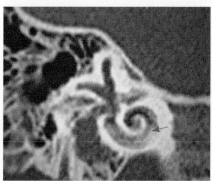

Fig. 5.5 HRCT temporal bone, bone window, oblique sagittal reconstruction image showing LO stage IIIa with ossification (red arrow) more than 180 degrees but less than 360 degrees in the basal turn.

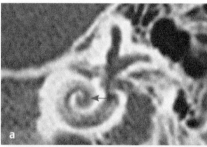

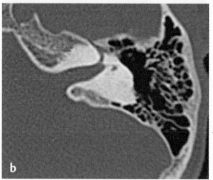

Fig. 5.6 HRCT temporal bone, bone window showing LO stage IIIb in, **(a)** oblique sagittal reconstruction image showing ossification (red arrow) more than 360 degrees in the basal turn and **(b)** complete LO of the inner ear ("white-out cochlea").

These drill-out procedures can be performed via standard mastoi-dectomy posterior tympanotomy approach or via an extended posterior tympanotomy approach for better access to the round window niche. In cases of LO, round window membrane appears as crystalline and white in color instead of dark gray color intraoperatively.

Depending on the extent and site of ossification, various types of entry into the cochlea can be done as depicted in **Fig. 5.7**.

Different surgical approaches as per the stage of ossification can be as follows:

1. Stage I: When the site of LO is confined to the round window, a separate cochleostomy can be done to gain access for electrode array insertion during CI (**Fig. 5.8**).
2. Stage II: When the ossification involves inferior turn of the basal turn, various options available are partial drill-out of the scala tympani of basal turn, which can be done via drilling of the round window or a separate cochleostomy, until the patency of cochlear lumen with access for electrode array insertion is attained (**Fig. 5.9**).
3. Stage IIIa: When the ossification involves more than 180 degrees but less than 360 degrees of basal turn (**Fig. 5.10**). Surgical options include:

   – Scala vestibuli insertion is considered for electrode array insertion if the ossification is confined to the scala tympani of the basal turn of cochlea (**Fig. 5.10a, b**).

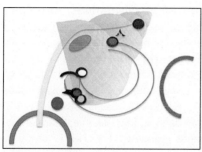

Fig. 5.7 Line diagram showing various sites of cochlear entry in cases of **labyrinthitis ossificans**. (■ light blue) round window, (■ pink) extended cochleostomy, (■ green) separate cochleostomy, (□ white) scala vestibuli insertion anterosuperior to round window, (■ orange) middle turn cochleostomy anterior to oval window and inferior to processus cochleariformis, (■ purple) apical turn cochleostomy just inferior to geniculate ganglion, (■ dark green) oval window, (■ dark blue) jugular bulb, (■ red) internal carotid artery, (■ yellow) facial nerve, (■ grey) hypotympanic cells and subcochlear canaliculus. The cochlea is being represented by a blurred shell of a snail.

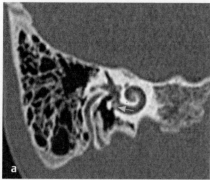

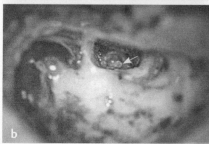

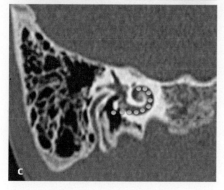

Fig. 5.8 HRCT temporal bone, bone window, oblique sagittal reconstruction images showing **labyrinthitis ossificans** stage 1: **(a)** ossification (green arrow) confined to the round window region, **(b)** crystalline white appearance of ossification intraoperatively (yellow arrow), and **(c)** schematic representation of electrode array (blue) insertion via anteroinferior cochleostomy.

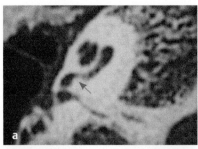

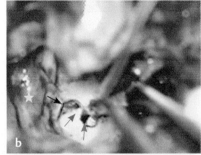

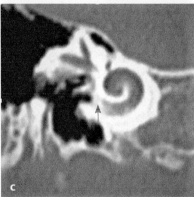

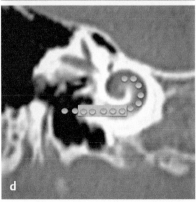

Fig. 5.9 Labyrinthitis ossificans stage II ossification (red arrow): **(a)** HRCT temporal bone, bone window axial section; **(b)** intraoperative image of a patient undergoing subtotal petrosectomy and cochlear implant (blue arrow) separate cochleostomy, (yellow star) dehiscent facial nerve, (black arrow) round window; **(c)** HRCT temporal bone, bone window, oblique sagittal reconstruction section; **(d)** schematic representation of electrode array (blue) insertion via separate cochleostomy and partial drill out of basal turn. *(Continued)*

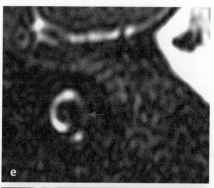

Fig. 5.9 *(Continued)* **(e)** MRI T2W CISS sequence coronal sections showing loss of fluid signal; **(f)** 3D reconstruction image of MRI showing loss of fluid signal in scala vestibuli of basal turn.

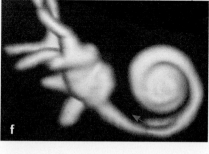

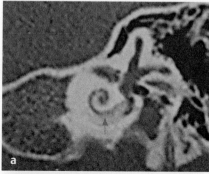

Fig. 5.10 Labyrinthitis ossificans stage IIIa, ossification (red arrow): **(a)** HRCT temporal bone, bone window, oblique sagittal reconstruction section, showing ossification of scala tympani with patent scala vestibuli; **(b)** schematic representation of electrode array (blue) insertion into scala vestibuli. *(Continued)*

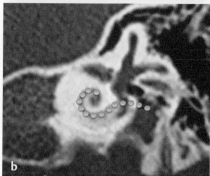

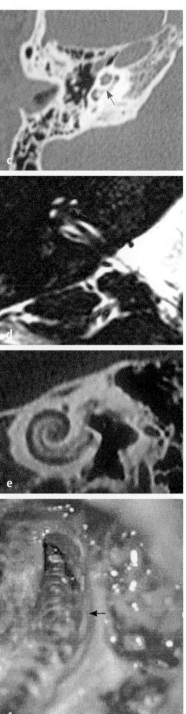

Fig. 5.10 *(Continued)* **(c)** HRCT temporal bone, bone window, axial section showing ossification in the basal turn; **(d)** MRI T2W CISS sequence axial section showing loss of fluid signal; **(e)** HRCT temporal bone, bone window, oblique sagittal reconstruction section, showing ossification of scala tympani with patent scala tympani; **(f)** intraoperative image showing partial drill out of basal turn with electrode array insertion (black arrow).

- Rarely, the ossification can involve only scala vestibuli and scala tympani is fortunately available for electrode array insertion (**Fig. 5.10c**).
- A complete drill-out of basal turn is the next option available if the ossification involves both scala tympani and scala vestibuli. Complete basal turn drill-out was first described by Cohen and Waltzman. If after the drill-out of the inferior part of the basal turn the ascending part is accessible, regular electrodes can be inserted (**Fig. 5.10f**). If in case the ascending part is not accessible, the next viable option available is the middle turn cochleostomy.

  Note: During complete drill-out of the basal turn, while going anterior, even if minimal bleeding is encountered while drilling, it indicates vasa vasorum of the internal carotid artery. Care must be taken to avoid drilling beyond 8 mm anterior as this may injure the carotid artery.

- Middle turn cochleostomy (**Fig. 5.11**) with an anterograde or a retrograde electrode array insertion is considered when the ascending segment of the basal turn is not accessible even after complete basal turn drill-out. Middle turn cochleostomy is usually done 2 mm anterior to the oval window, just inferior to the processus cochleariformis (**Fig. 5.11b, c**). For doing middle turn cochleostomy, the majority of otologists remove the incus bar and perform an extended posterior tympanotomy with removal of the incus. The authors, however, prefer to do this cochleostomy without completely removing the incus bar or incus. Only if the visualization is poor do they recommend these two extensions. Double array/split array with two shorter electrode arrays with around 10 electrodes each was used in the past but is not available at present. Compressed arrays can be used in such cases. The retrograde electrode array insertion will require reprogramming of the electrodes by the audiologist for better speech perception.

4. Stage IIIB: When the ossification involves more than 360 degrees of the basal turn (**Fig. 5.12**), total drill-out of basal and middle turn or a circummodiolar drill-out of cochlea is done by creating a trough around the modiolus. The risks during this procedure are damage to the modiolus, labyrinthine part of the facial nerve, and damage to the carotid artery. A better option in many of these cases could be an auditory brainstem implant.

Sometimes due to financial constraints, it may not be possible to arrange for funds for a CI. Kirtane et al[18] suggested that early stenting of the cochlear lumen with sterile nonfunctional dummy electrode array (depth gauge) can keep the lumen patent and prevent further ossification (cochlear stenting). Later, once the funds for CI have been arranged, the stent can be removed leaving the fibrous sheath at the cochleostomy and the functioning implant electrode can be inserted through this sheath. This is an off-label use of depth gauge.

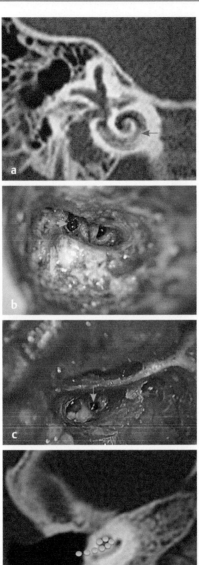

Fig. 5.11 LO stage IIIa ossification (red arrow), **(a)** HRCT temporal bone, bone window, oblique sagittal reconstruction section, showing ossification more than 180 degrees but less than 360 degrees in the basal turn of cochlea, **(b)** middle turn cochleostomy via extended posterior tympanotomy approach with removal of incus bar and incus, **(c)** middle turn cochleostomy (blue arrow) via posterior tympanotomy approach with preservation of incus bar (yellow) and incus, **(d)** schematic representation of electrode array (blue) insertion via middle turn cochleostomy.

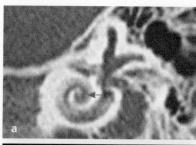

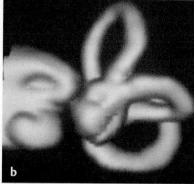

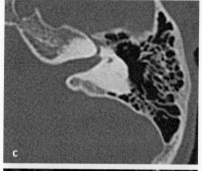

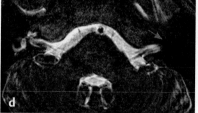

Fig. 5.12 Labyrinthitis ossificans (LO) stage IIIb ossification (red arrow): **(a)** HRCT temporal bone, bone window, oblique sagittal reconstruction section, showing ossification more than 360 degrees in the basal turn of cochlea; **(b)** 3D reconstruction image showing loss of fluid signal in the cochlea; **(c)** HRCT temporal bone, bone window, axial sections showing complete LO of the inner ear ("white-out cochlea"); **(d)** MRI CISS/FIESTA sequence, axial section showing complete loss of fluid signal in the cochlea.

Otosclerosis

Hearing loss due to otosclerosis may be conductive due to fenestral otosclerosis (stapes fixation) and mixed or pure sensorineural hearing loss due to retrofenestral or far advanced otosclerosis. Otosclerosis is a form of osteodystrophy that mainly affects the otic capsule. It is mostly autosomal dominant and more commonly affects females. The main pathophysiology involved with otosclerosis includes osteolysis (due to increased osteoclastic activity) followed by osteogenesis, which shows classical histological findings of vascular proliferation, bone resorption, and formation of connective tissue stroma. The active form of otosclerosis is known as otospongiosis. Sensorineural hearing loss in otosclerosis is probably due to the lytic enzymes that are released from otosclerotic foci into the perilymph[19] or due to narrowing of the cochlear lumen which leads to distortion of the basilar membrane.[20] In the active vascular phase (otospongiosis), the normal lamellar bone is resorbed and is replaced by thick, irregular bone (sclerotic phase) as the disease progresses. The most common site of otosclerotic foci is the fissula ante fenestrum, however, in 10% of the cases, the sensorineural hearing loss may be retrofenetral involving the endosteum caused due to narrowing of the basal turn.

HRCT temporal bone is at present the imaging modality of choice to detect the foci of demineralization within the otic capsule in otosclerosis. On HRCT, the findings can be:

1. In fenestral otospongiotic lesions, the margin of the oval window appears wider than normal due to increased areas of decalcification, whereas mature osteosclerotic foci makes the oval window area narrow.
2. Resorbed bone appears as areas of radiolucent zones with decreased density (**Fig. 5.13**).
3. "Double-ring" or "halo effect" is a typical sign of otospongiosis seen in retrofenestral otosclerosis and represents the pericochlear confluent foci surrounding the cochlear lumen[21] (**Fig. 5.13a**).
4. Narrowing and scalloping with irregularities of the cochlear turns are seen due to sclerotic foci and are mainly seen at the basal turn of cochlea[22] (**Fig. 5.13b**).

Active disease may also be identified on MRI. An active retrofenestral disease will be seen as a ring of intermediate signal in the pericochlear and perilabyrinthine regions on T1W MRI with contrast[23] (**Fig. 5.14**). This occurs due to the pooling of contrast (gadolinium) into the vascular foci, and is seen as a mild to moderate enhancement on T1W MRI with contrast.

The severity of disease on HRCT has been correlated to the degree of sensorineural hearing loss. Various classifications have been put forward for otosclerosis, initially by Valvassori, later by Rotteveel and Symons and Fanning. The classification by Symons and Fannings is widely accepted and commonly followed.

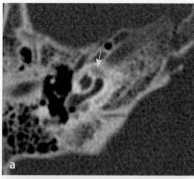

Fig. 5.13 HRCT temporal bone, bone window shows retrofenestral otosclerosis: **(a)** radiolucent areas (yellow arrow) on axial sections with a double halo appearance, and **(b)** radiolucent areas (yellow arrow) with narrowing of basal turn (pink arrow) on coronal sections.

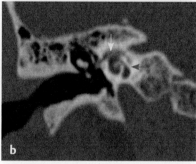

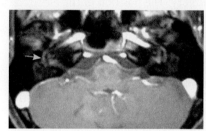

Fig. 5.14 MRI T1W with contrast, axial section shows enhancement (green arrow) in the pericochlear and perilabyrinthine region in retrofenestral otosclerosis.

Valvassori[21] characterized the otosclerotic lesions by hypodensity of the otic capsule or footplate thickening into four categories:

1. Anterior (fenestral) focus.
2. Pericochlear focus without endosteal extension.
3. Pericochlear focus with endosteal extension.
4. Pericochlear focus and footplate thickening.

Rotteveel Classification[24]

- Type 1: Solely fenestral otosclerosis (thickened footplate and/or narrowed or enlarged windows).
- Type 2: Retrofenestral with or without fenestral involvement:
  - Type 2a: Double ring effect.

- Type 2b: Narrowed basal turn.
- Type 2c: Double ring effect and narrowed basal turn.

• Type 3: Severe retrofenestral otosclerosis (unrecognizable otic capsule) with or without fenestral involvement.

Symons and Fanning[25] Classification of Otosclerosis

- Grade 0: Normal (**Fig. 5.15a**).
- Grade 1: Solely fenestral otosclerosis (**Fig. 5.15b**).
- Grade 2: Patchy localized retrofenestral disease with or without fenestral involvement:

   - Grade 2a Basal cochlear (**Fig. 5.15c**).
   - Grade 2b: Apical or midcochlear (**Fig. 5.15d**).
   - Grade 2c: Basal cochlear with apical or middle turn involvement (**Fig. 5.15e**).

- Grade 3: Diffuse confluent retrofenestral involvement with or without fenestral involvement (**Fig. 5.15f**).

CI is the treatment of choice in patients with far advanced otosclerosis. CI is highly challenging in patients with otosclerosis as there is a high chance of misplacement of the electrode array, facial nerve stimulation (FNS), and thus increased possibility of revision surgery. The position of the electrode array plays an important role in deciding the outcome of CI. Electrode insertion can be difficult because of the presence of cochlear ossification or pericochlear hypodensity leading to misplacement.

Several studies have mentioned the high incidence of FNS in CI for far advanced otosclerosis, and this being one of the major reasons for device explantation in such patients. The incidence of FNS reported in the literature varies from 0.9[26] to 14.6%.[27] FNS occurs due to decreased electrical impedance of the altered bone of the otic capsule thus causing the spread of current from the electrode to the facial nerve or due to the reduction of distance between the facial nerve and electrode due to the presence of lucent areas. Most frequent FNS is seen in the superior part of the basal turn or the middle turn of the cochlea where the labyrinthine segment and the geniculate ganglion are the closest. The distance between the labyrinthine segment of the facial nerve and the basal turn of the cochlea is the thinnest and is 0.52 mm (Kelsall et al).[28] A higher threshold of stimulation needs to be avoided, as there can be spread of electric current from the otosclerotic bone to the surrounding structures, which can not only cause FNS but also vestibular stimulation. In far advanced otosclerosis, perimodiolar or modiolar hugging electrode arrays (half banded) are preferred as low current threshold levels are enough to stimulate spiral ganglion cells thus preventing the spread of current to the adjacent vital structures. Also, the current is directed toward the modiolus and not the lateral wall. Lateral wall electrodes are preferably avoided to prevent FNS, due to proximity of the middle turn of cochlea to the labyrinthine segment of the facial nerve (**Fig. 5.16**).

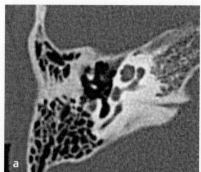

Fig. 5.15 HRCT temporal bone, axial sections, bone window showing grading of otosclerosis (red arrow): **(a)** grade 0 (normal), **(b)** grade 1 (solely fenestral), **(c)** grade 2a (basal turn), **(d)** grade 2b (apical or middle turn). *(Continued)*

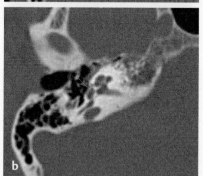

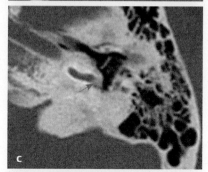

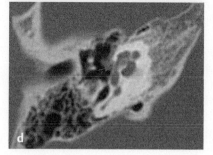

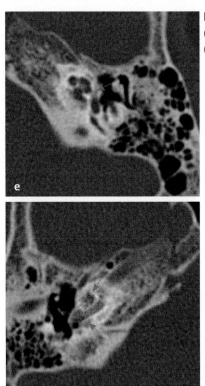

Fig. 5.15 *(Continued)* **(e)** grade 2c (basal and middle turn), and **(f)** grade 3 (diffuse confluent).

Temporal Bone Trauma

Trauma to the temporal bone can lead to hearing loss. This can be due to labyrinthine concussion or temporal bone fracture (transverse/otic capsule involving). Trauma may lead to degeneration of hair cells, supporting cells, and/or ganglion cells. As time progresses, it may lead to fibrosis and ossification in the labyrinth. In radiology, therefore, HRCT temporal bone of a recent temporal bone fracture might show a fracture line running through the labyrinth, pneumolabyrinth and haziness in the middle ear due to hemorrhage (**Fig. 5.17a**). With time, an old fracture line would show signs of healing with ossification in cochlea (**Fig. 5.17b**). This ossification usually affects scala tympani of basal turn. Therefore an early cochlear implantation should be planned in such patients. Proper evaluation is important if the fracture seems to be involving internal acoustic canal (IAC) as it may rarely lead to cochlear nerve transection. Complications associated with cochlear implantation post trauma include incomplete electrode insertion due to ossification/fibrosis, CSF leak, and FNS.

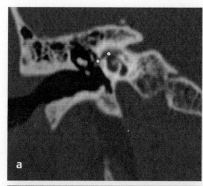
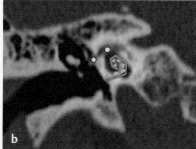
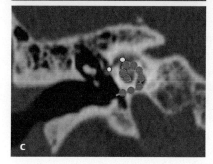

Fig. 5.16 HRCT temporal bone, coronal sections, bone window showing retrofenestral otosclerosis: **(a)** proximity of labyrinthine segment (yellow) of the facial nerve to the middle turn of the cochlea with otosclerotic focus in between. **(b)** Schematic representation of use of half banded modiolus hugging electrode array (pink) with electrodes (light blue) away from facial nerve, thus avoiding **facial nerve stimulation** (FNS). **(c)** Schematic representation of use of full banded lateral wall electrode array (pink) with electrodes (dark blue) close to the labyrinthine segment of facial nerve (yellow) and circumferential spread of current causing FNS. Lateral wall electrode arrays are preferably avoided in cases of retrofenestral otosclerosis to avoid FNS.

Paget's Disease

Paget's disease (osteitis deformans) is a common bone disorder of unresolved etiology characterized by excessive bone resorption by osteoclasts followed by an increase in new and abnormal bone formation by osteoblasts. If the skull is affected, particularly the temporal bones, then it may result in hearing loss and eventually develop into profound deafness. The prevalence of hearing loss has been estimated to range from 30 to 50% in all patients evaluated with Paget's disease of the skull.[29,30] Hearing loss in Paget's disease of the skull may be conductive, sensorineural, or mixed. The mechanism of sensorineural hearing loss may be related to

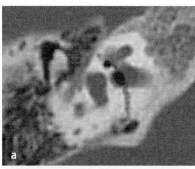

Fig. 5.17 HRCT temporal bone, axial section, bone window showing **(a)** recent transverse fracture passing through the otic capsule with pneumolabyrinth in cochlea and internal acoustic canal with haziness in middle ear cleft due to hemorrhage, **(b)** old transverse fracture passing through the otic capsule showing signs of healing and ossification in the middle turn of the cochlea.

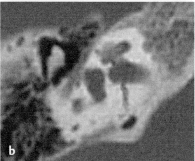

loss of bone mineral density in the cochlear capsule,[31] hair cell damage,[32] and progressive internal auditory canal stenosis with compression of the eighth cranial nerve.[33] The radiology findings on HRCT temporal bone reveal homogeneously diffuse hyperostosis of the skull and a slight loss of bone mineral density in the cochlear capsule (**Fig. 5.18**).

The side of surgery is chosen on the basis of better patent IAC. During surgery, Takano et al[34] found that intraoperatively there was masked osteolysis of the otic capsule, and the bones surrounding the semicircular canals were completely resorbed and replaced by perilymph-like substance. They also reported that the bone surrounding the cochlea along the facial canal appeared transparent. The bone was extremely fragile.

Langerhans Cell Histiocytosis

Langerhans cell histiocytosis (LCH) is a rare disease of unknown etiology, characterized by abnormal polyclonal proliferation of Langerhans cells, leading to local tissue invasion and destruction. The temporal bone is involved in 19 to 25% of cases.[35] The common otologic symptoms are otorrhea, soft-tissue swelling, and hearing loss. The hearing loss is usually conductive and secondary to middle ear soft-tissue infiltration, ossicular erosion, or aural polyps. Sensorineural hearing loss and facial paresis are rare.

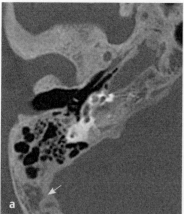

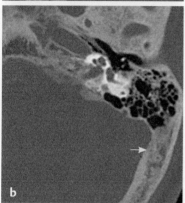

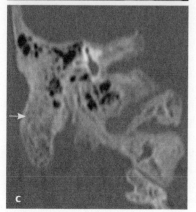

Fig. 5.18 HRCT temporal bone, bone window shows Paget's disease with diffuse hyperostosis (yellow arrow) of the skull and loss of mineral bone density (red arrow) in the cochlear capsule on **(a, b)** axial sections and **(c, d)** coronal sections. *(Continued)*

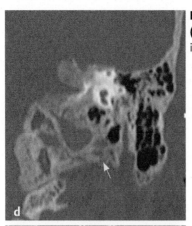

Fig. 5.18   *(Continued)* **(d)** coronal sections. **(e)** axial sections showing obliteration of internal acoustic canal.

Radiological findings of LCH involving temporal bones usually show extensive destruction of the temporal bone involving the mastoid, with the squamous part and the middle ear being less affected.[36,37] The lesions have indistinct margins, and the smaller structures of the bony labyrinth and auditory ossicle chain may show erosion. However, involvement of the auditory ossicles and the internal ear is not as frequent as might be expected from the extensive bony damage usually seen. In many patients, CT shows associated enhanced soft-tissue masses that occasionally had extradural extension. On MRI, these masses show a strong signal intensity on T2W imaging and variable signal intensity (low to high) on T1W imaging, often with edema or inflammation around the lesion[38,39] and with marked enhancement after administration of gadolinium.

There is very limited literature on cochlear implantation in LCH. Case report by Gupta et al[40] mentioned that surgery was done when the patient was in remission 2 years after chemotherapy. During surgery, cochleostomy was performed anteroinferior to the round window niche. The bone was found to be thickened and hard with fibrous tissue in the basal turn of the cochlea. The HRCT temporal images of the patient are being shared here with permission from the authors (**Fig. 5.19**).

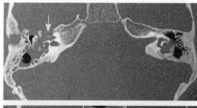

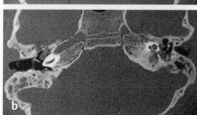

Fig. 5.19 HRCT temporal bone, bone window shows Langerhans cell histiocytosis: **(a)** lytic lesions (yellow arrow) seen involving the labyrinth on coronal section, **(b)** resolution (red arrow) of lytic lesions after completion of chemotherapy. Patient underwent a cochlear implant on the right side. (Reproduced with permission from Gupta et al)[40]

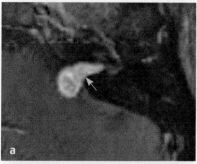

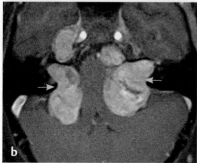

Fig. 5.20 MRI brain with contrast showing vestibular schwannoma with classical ice cream cone appearance (green arrow) in axial sections, **(a)** unilateral, **(b)** a patient of neurofibromatosis 2 presenting with bilateral vestibular schwannomas.

Cerebellopontine Angle Lesions

Acoustic Neuroma

Till sometime back, presence of acoustic neuroma was considered to be a contraindication for CI. However for the past few years, there have been multiple papers on CI in acoustic neuromas. Most acoustic neuromas have an intracanalicular component which widens the porus of IAC (**Fig. 5.20**).

Usually, it remains away from the cochlea, however rarely it may grow laterally, transmodiolar or transmacular into cochlea or vestibule, respectively. Involvement of fundus of IAC is associated with higher rates of hearing loss and lesser chances of preserving the cochlear nerve intraoperatively. Rarely, we can find intralabyrinthine schwannomas too where patients may present with vertigo, tinnitus, and/or hearing loss (**Fig. 5.21**).

We also need to remember that even after CI, these patients may need regular follow-ups with MR scans for their cerebellopontine (CP) angle pathology, therefore an implant with higher MRI compatibility with option of magnet removal (to have lesser artifacts) would be the most appropriate.

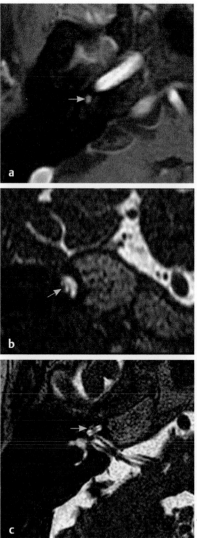

Fig. 5.21 MRI brain shows cochlear schwannoma (green arrow) involving the apical turn, **(a)** enhancement seen in the coronal sections on T1W with contrast, **(b)** loss of fluid signal on coronal section in T2W, and **(c)** loss of fluid signal on axial section in T2W.

Arachnoid Cyst

Arachnoid cysts are cysts filled with CSF covered by arachnoid cells. They develop at the base of the skull, the surface of the brain, or on the arachnoid membrane.

Most arachnoid cysts are located in the middle cranial fossa. Localizations in the posterior fossa, the CP angle, and the cerebellar hemispheres are rare.

They appear as hyperintense cystic spaces on T2W MR images (**Fig. 5.22**). Most cases are incidental imaging findings while symptomatic lesions may present with headache, seizure, or focal neurological deficit. Arachnoid cysts are usually asymptomatic and conservative management with regular follow-up based on radiological evaluation is sufficient. Surgical indications include rapidly growing cysts, compression and displacement of the surrounding neurovascular structures, and symptomatic patients. The surgical procedures include drainage, total or partial removal of the cyst, shunting, or fistulization of the cyst to the subarachnoid space. Usually, CI can be done safely in these patients with or without surgery for the cyst per se.

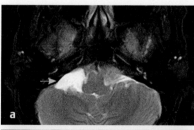
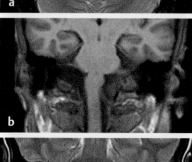
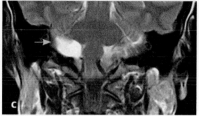

Fig. 5.22 MRI brain shows arachnoid cyst (green arrow) at CP angle on right side which appears hyperintense on T2W and no signal on T1W images: **(a)** T2W axial section, **(b)** T1W coronal sections, and **(c)** T2W coronal sections.

Meningioma

The second most common lesion in the CP angle is meningioma which accounts for 10 to 15% of cases. Meningiomas that extend into the IAC are very rare and present with symptoms similar to vestibular schwannoma such as unilateral sensorineural hearing loss, tinnitus, and vertigo, if there is compression of the cochlear or the vestibular nerves. Meningiomas arise from the arachnoid meningothelial cells and thus show a classical "dural tail" sign on MRI, which represents the enhancement of the nonneoplastic thickened peritumoral dura. They show homogenous enhancement on T1W MRI with contrast and are isointense on a T1W and T2W MRI. Meningiomas typically have a broad base at their origin and a hemispheric shape on the opposite side (**Fig. 5.23**). As mentioned above in vestibular schwannoma, repeated MRI may be required in cases of meningioma. If the patient undergoes CI, care must be taken to consider for a better MRI compatibility device with the option of magnet removal.

TORCH Complex Infections

TORCH infections include toxoplasmosis, rubella, cytomegalovirus (CMV), and herpes simplex. CMV is the most common nongenetic cause of sensorineural hearing loss. The risk of congenital hearing loss due to an infective cause is largely dependent on socioeconomic status (congenital CMV infection), availability of prevention strategies such as vaccination (congenital rubella), or hygienic measures (congenital toxoplasmosis). The mode of transmission of these infections can be in utero (transplacental as

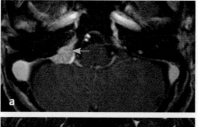
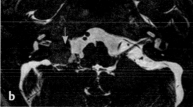

Fig. 5.23 MRI brain shows meningioma (green arrows) at CP angle on the right side which appears hyperintense on T1W with contrast with a "dural tail" and isointense on T2W images on axial sections **(a)** T1W with contrast and **(b)** T2W.

in CMV) or intrapartum. CMV and rubella cause extensive damage during the first trimester whereas toxoplasmosis effects in the third trimester. CMV causes viral labyrinthitis and inflammation causing cochlear damage. Rubella virus causes direct damage and cell death in the organ of Corti and stria vascularis.

CMV along with cochlear deafness is characterized by chorioretinitis, optic nerve atrophy, and microcephaly. Congenital rubella syndrome manifests as hearing loss, congenital cataracts, microcephaly, mental retardation, thrombocytopenia, cardiac anomalies, and a characteristic blueberry muffin rash. Congenital toxoplasmosis is characterized by microcephaly, intracerebral calcifications, and chorioretinitis. Lately zika virus infection has been identified as a major cause of fetal injury and newborn disability that can cause congenital hearing loss.

In CMV, the CT brain may show intracranial calcifications in the periventricular regions and basal ganglia. Other characteristics include hypodense areas in the white matter, ventriculomegaly, cerebral atrophy, and destructive encephalopathy. Characteristic features on the MRI brain include microcephaly, periventricular calcifications, and subependymal cysts (**Fig. 5.24**) representing focal areas of necrosis in the white matter, ventriculomegaly, subarachnoid space enlargement, and delayed myelination.

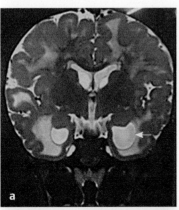
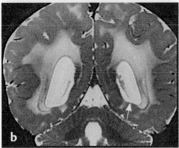

Fig. 5.24 MRI Brain in congenital CMV infection showing **(a, b, c, d)** subependymal cyst (yellow arrow) and **(e, f)** hyperintensities in the periventricular white matter region.

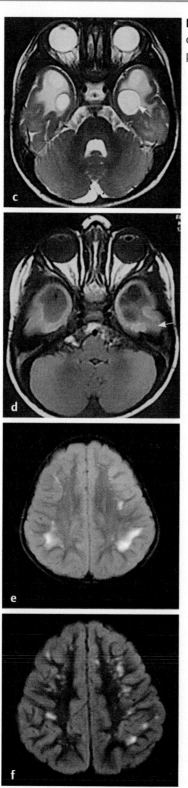

Fig. 5.24 *(Continued)* **(c, d)** subependymal cyst and **(e, f)** hyperintensities in the periventricular white matter region.

In congenital rubella syndrome, microcephaly and vasculitis are commonly seen. There are extensive degenerative arterial changes that occur leading to small loci of necrosis which are clearly seen on MRI.

References

1. Hoffman RA, Brookler KH, Bergeron RT. Radiologic diagnosis of labyrinthitis ossificans. Ann Otol Rhinol Laryngol 197988(2 Pt 1):253–257
2. Suga F, Lindsay JR. Labyrinthitis ossificans. Ann Otol Rhinol Laryngol 1977;86(1 Pt 1): 17–29
3. Paparella MM, Sugiura S. The pathology of suppurative labyrinthitis. Ann Otol Rhinol Laryngol 1967;76(3):554–586
4. Balkany T, Gantz B, Nadol JB Jr. Multichannel cochlear implants in partially ossified cochleas. Ann Otol Rhinol Laryngol Suppl 1988;135(5, suppl2)3–7
5. Gantz BJ, McCabe BF, Tyler RS. Use of multichannel cochlear implants in obstructed and obliterated cochleas. Otolaryngol Head Neck Surg 1988;98(1):72–81
6. Sanna M, Free RH, Falcioni M, Merkus P. Surgery for cochlear and other auditory implants. Thieme; 2016
7. Swartz JD, Mandell DM, Faerber EN, et al. Labyrinthine ossification: etiologies and CT findings. Radiology 1985;157(2):395–398
8. Weissman JL, Kamerer DB. Labyrinthitis ossificans. Am J Otolaryngol 1993;14(5): 363–365
9. Chan CC, Saunders DE, Chong WK, Hartley BE, Raglan E, Rajput K. Advancement in post-meningitic lateral semicircular canal labyrinthitis ossificans. J Laryngol Otol 2007;121(2):105–109
10. Balkany TJ, Dreisbach JN, Seibert CE. Radiographic imaging of the cochlear implant candidate: preliminary results. Otolaryngol Head Neck Surg 1986;95(5):592–597
11. Smullen JL, Balkany TJ. Implantation of the ossified cochlea. Oper Tech Otolaryngol– Head Neck Surg 2005;16(2):117–120
12. Balkany T, Gantz BJ, Steenerson RL, Cohen NL. Systematic approach to electrode insertion in the ossified cochlea. Otolaryngol Head Neck Surg 1996;114(1):4–11
13. Hohman MH, Backous DD. Techniques for cochlear implant electrode placement in the ossified cochlea. Oper Tech Otolaryngol–Head Neck Surg 2010;21(4):239–242
14. Millar DA, Hillman TA, Shelton C. Implantation of the ossified cochlea: management with the split electrode array. Laryngoscope 2005;115(12):2155–2160
15. Roland JTJ Jr, Coelho DH, Pantelides H, Waltzman SB. Partial and double-array implantation of the ossified cochlea. Otol Neurotol 2008;29(8):1068–1075
16. Bauer PW, Roland PS. Clinical results with the Med-El compressed and split arrays in the United States. Laryngoscope 2004;114(3):428–433
17. Bredberg G, Lindström B, Löppönen H, Skarzynski H, Hyodo M, Sato H. Electrodes for ossified cochleas. Am J Otol 1997;18(6, Suppl)S42–S43
18. Kirtane MV, More YI, Mankekar G. Cochlear stenting: how I do it. Eur Arch Otorhinolaryngol 2010;267(6):985–987
19. Linthicum FH Jr. Histopathology of otosclerosis. Otolaryngol Clin North Am 1993;26(3):335–352
20. Linthicum FH Jr, Filipo R, Brody S. Sensorineural hearing loss due to cochlear otospongiosis: theoretical considerations of etiology. Ann Otol Rhinol Laryngol 1975;84(4 Pt 1):544–551
21. Valvassori GE. Imaging of otosclerosis. Otolaryngol Clin North Am 1993;26(3):359–371
22. Swartz JD, Mandell DW, Berman SE, Wolfson RJ, Marlowe FI, Popky GL. Cochlear otosclerosis (otospongiosis): CT analysis with audiometric correlation. Radiology 1985;155(1):147–150

23. Purohit B, Op de Beeck K, Hermans R. Role of MRI as first-line modality in the detection of previously undiagnosed otosclerosis: a single tertiary institute experience. Insights Imaging 2020;11(1):71

24. Rotteveel LJC, Proops DW, Ramsden RT, Saeed SR, van Olphen AF, Mylanus EAM. Cochlear implantation in 53 patients with otosclerosis: demographics, computed tomographic scanning, surgery, and complications. Otol Neurotol 2004;25(6):943–952

25. Marshall AH, Fanning N, Symons S, Shipp D, Chen JM, Nedzelski JM. Cochlear implantation in cochlear otosclerosis. Laryngoscope 2005;115(10):1728–1733

26. Lindsay JR. Histopathology of otosclerosis. Arch Otolaryngol 1973;97(1):24–29

27. Niparko JK, Oviatt DL, Coker NJ, Sutton L, Waltzman SB, Cohen NL; VA Cooperative Study Group on Cochlear Implantation. Facial nerve stimulation with cochlear implantation. Otolaryngol Head Neck Surg 1991;104(6):826–830

28. Kelsall DC, Shallop JK, Brammeier TG, Prenger EC. Facial nerve stimulation after Nucleus 22-channel cochlear implantation. Am J Otol 1997;18(3):336–341

29. Avioli LV. Paget's disease: state of the art. Clin Ther 1987;9(6):567–576

30. Nager GT. Paget's disease of the temporal bone. Ann Otol Rhinol Laryngol 1975;84(4 Pt 3, Suppl 22)1–32

31. Monsell EM, Cody DD, Bone HG, et al. Hearing loss in Paget's disease of bone: the relationship between pure-tone thresholds and mineral density of the cochlear capsule. Hear Res 1995;83(1-2):114–120

32. Lenarz T, Hoth S, Frank K, Ziegler R. [Hearing disorders in Paget's disease]. Laryngol Rhinol Otol (Stuttg) 1986;65(4):213–217

33. Ginsberg LE, Elster AD, Moody DM. MRI of Paget disease with temporal bone involvement presenting with sensorineural hearing loss. J Comput Assist Tomogr 1992;16(2):314–316

34. Takano K, Saikawa E, Ogasawara N, Himi T. Cochlear implantation in a patient with Paget's disease. Am J Otolaryngol 2014;35(3):408–410

35. Martini A, Aimoni C, Trevisani M, Marangoni P. Langerhans' cell histiocytosis: report of a case with temporal localization. Int J Pediatr Otorhinolaryngol 2000;55(1):51–56

36. Cunningham MJ, Curtin HD, Butkiewicz BL. Histiocytosis X of the temporal bone: CT findings. J Comput Assist Tomogr 1988;12(1):70–74

37. Hadjigeorgi C, Parpounas C, Zarmakoupis P, Lafoyianni S. Eosinophilic granuloma of the temporal bone: radiological approach in the pediatric patient. Pediatr Radiol 1990;20(7):546–549

38. Hermans R, De Foer B, Smet M-H, et al. Eosinophilic granuloma of the head and neck: CT and MRI features in three cases. Pediatr Radiol 1994;24(1):33–36

39. Beltran J, Aparisi F, Bonmati LM, Rosenberg ZS, Present D, Steiner GC. Eosinophilic granuloma: MRI manifestations. Skeletal Radiol 1993;22(3):157–161

40. Gupta G, Jain A, Grover M. Successful cochlear implantation in Langerhans cell histiocytosis: a rare case. Cochlear Implants Int 2018;19(2):115–118

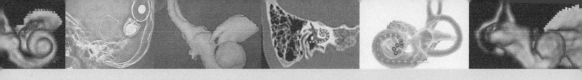

Chapter 6

Intraoperative and Postoperative Radiology Including Complications

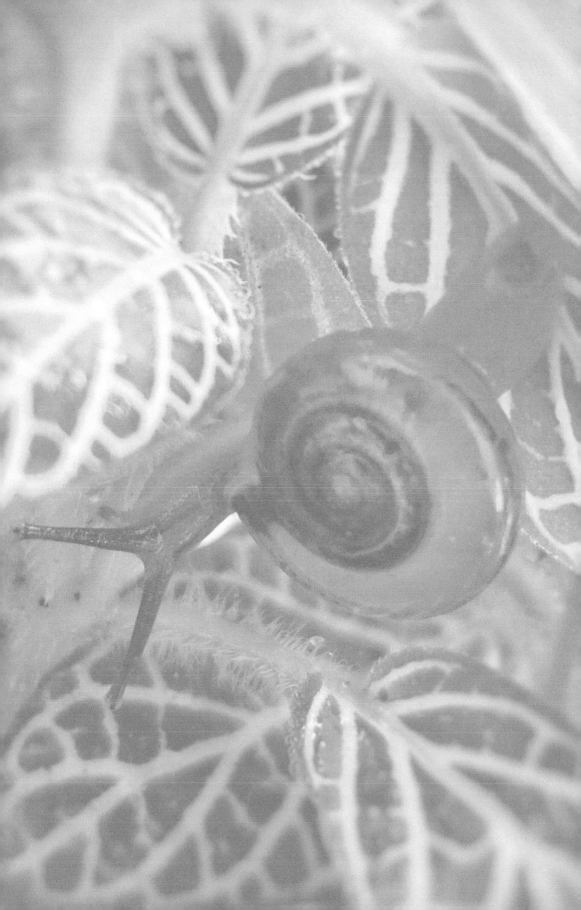

6 Intraoperative and Postoperative Radiology Including Complications

Introduction

Radiology is an important part of cochlear implantation, be it for preoperative evaluation or intra/postoperative confirmation of implant placement. For the latter, in the majority of cases, only a plain radiograph is enough and advanced modality is rarely needed. In fact advanced modalities may have their inherent disadvantages, such as radiation exposure with computed tomography (CT) and artifacts and risk of implant migration with magnetic resonance imaging (MRI). Though, with advances in technology (of CT/MRI machines and cochlear implants [CI]), these problems have been negated to some extent, still plain radiograph suffices in the majority of cases.

Why is it Needed?

Intraoperative/postoperative radiology helps to confirm the correct placement of the electrode array. Many times it is also important medicolegally. With the help of intraoperative electrically evoked compound action potential (ECAP) measurements, the position of the electrode array can be confirmed in the majority of cases. However, in certain conditions, intraoperative ECAP measurements may not give us a true picture, viz malformed cochlea, ossified cochlea, revision surgeries, misplaced electrode array into the vestibule, and tip fold overs. A radiograph also serves as a reference for future evaluation like in cases of electrode migration.

Various imaging modalities available for intraoperative and post-operative radiology include:

1. Portable plain X-ray film radiography.
2. C-arm fluoroscopy.
3. Cone-beam CT.
4. Digital volume tomography.
5. Intraoperative fluoroscopy.
6. Navigation-based/computer-assisted CI surgery.

Plain X-ray film radiography and cone-beam CT are discussed in this chapter, and rest will be discussed in detail in the next chapter on recent advances.

Plain X-ray Film Radiography

Imaging with high-resolution CT (HRCT) and MRI has largely replaced the use of conventional radiographs in the field of otology in detecting various temporal bone pathologies. Postoperative imaging after cochlear implantation is usually performed by conventional X-ray or by multislice CT (MSCT). Conventional X-ray is routinely used in children due to short investigation time, no need of sedation, and low radiation dose. Conventional X-ray are of great importance as the entire length of the electrode array, position and intracochlear placement of the electrode array, its integrity and depth of insertion can be well seen and analyzed. CT is not routinely recommended and is necessary only if complications arise. Though MSCT after cochlear implantation allows for three-dimensional imaging, it may unfortunately provide metal artifacts and thus individual electrodes cannot be clearly distinguished.

Several radiographic projections have been described for imaging in CI. The most used radiographic projections for intraoperative and postoperative assessment are lateral oblique and anteroposterior views. The Stenvers view and its variations are the best projections for demonstrating the position of intracochlear electrode arrays. Knowledge about the direction of the cochlea in the skull is of great importance to define the direction of X-ray projection. An optimum view and ideal radiograph of the intracochlear electrode array, located in the basal and middle turns around the modiolus of the cochlea, can be obtained if the central ray (CR) of X-rays is directed at the cochlea and is parallel to the modiolus (**Fig. 6.1**).

Points to be taken into consideration for better understanding of radiographic imaging, as shown in the figure, include:

1. Petrous pyramid is directed anteromedially.
2. Apex of the cochlea is directed anteriorly and laterally.

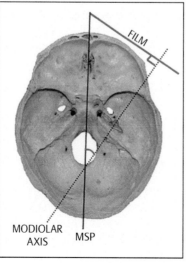

MODIOLAR AXIS   MSP   FILM

Fig. 6.1 Superior view of the base of the skull showing the measured angle between the mid sagittal plane (MSP, black line) and the long axis (black dotted line) of the cochlea (purple) to be 45 to 50 degrees.

3. The cochlear axis is perpendicular to the long axis of the petrous pyramid.
4. The cochlear axis makes an angle of usually 45 to 50 degrees with the midsagittal plane (MSP), so the head should be turned to such a degree, for a better view of the inner ear structures and the electrode array.
5. The three semicircular canals (SCCs) are perpendicular to each other.
6. The modiolar axis of the cochlea is parallel to the plane of the superior SCC.
7. The X-ray beam should be along the modiolar axis or axis of the superior SCC (SSCC).
8. The SSCC is perpendicular to the posterior wall of the petrous pyramid.
9. Frankfurt plane is a line through the infraorbital rim and superior aspect of the external auditory meatus and is also known as horizontal plane.

Lateral-Oblique Views

Stenvers View

1. Dr H.W. Stenver in 1917 described Stenvers view of the temporal bone.
2. It is an oblique posteroanterior radiographic projection of the petrous bone with the patient in the prone or sitting position.
3. The head is turned with the side being examined situated closest to the detector.
4. The head is adjusted such that the MSP is angled 45 degrees to the film plane (**Fig. 6.2**).
5. The infraorbitomeatal line is perpendicular to the plane of the film.
6. The central X-ray beam is angled 12 degrees cephalad to the infraorbitomeatal plane and centered on the occipital protuberance.
7. The entire petrous pyramid, arcuate eminence, porus acusticus, internal acoustic meatus, labyrinth with its vestibule, lateral, and superior SCC, cochlea and mastoid antrum can be visualized in this view.

Modified Stenvers View

1. It is an oblique posteroanterior view and was first described by Marsh.
2. Modified Stenvers view is the most commonly used radiographic method to assess CI electrode placement.
3. According to Marsh et al,[1] a view is considered optimum when the central X-ray beam is parallel to the modiolar axis so that the electrode array is essentially parallel to the film plane and electrode overlap does not affect quantification of insertion depth.

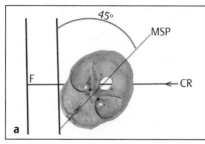

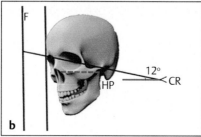

Fig. 6.2 (a, b) Stenvers view with head turned by 45 degrees and the CR angled at 12 degrees to the HP. (Dotted line MSP, midsagittal plane; CR, central ray; red dotted line HP, horizontal plane; F, film).

4. Various variations in the angle between the MSP and the plane of the X-ray film and the angle between the central X-ray beam and the horizontal plane have been mentioned in the study done by Marsh et al.[1]

5. The 50-degree angle between the MSP and the plane of the X-ray film and zero-degree angle between the central X-ray beam and the horizontal plane (referred to as 50/0) was considered the best and was later described by Xu et al[2] as the Cochlear view in his study.

6. The 50/0 degree oblique view of the petrous bone results in a radiograph that shows the SSCC as a vertical lucent line, the vestibule as an oval lucency, and the intracochlear electrode array located in basal and middle turn as a nonoverlapping spiral (**Fig. 6.3**).

Cochlear View

1. The cochlear view was described in detail by Xu et al.[2]

2. The patient is seated in front of a vertical device. The head rests on the forehead, nose, and zygomatic bone on the implanted side.

3. The MSP is then adjusted to form an angle of 50 degrees with the plane of the film and the infraorbitalmeatal plane is perpendicular to the X-ray film.

4. The CR penetrates the occiput without any angulation and exits from the skull at a point 3.0 cm anterior and 0.7 cm superior to the external auditory meatus closest to the image receptor.

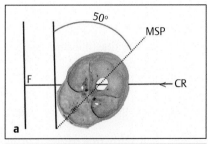

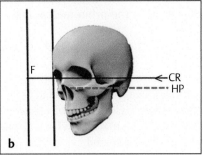

Fig. 6.3 (a, b) Modified Stenvers view with head turned by 50 degree and CR being parallel to HP. (Dotted line MSP, midsagittal plane; CR, central ray along the long axis of cochlea; red dotted line HP, horizontal plane; F, film).

Arcelin View

1. It is the exact opposite of Stenvers view.
2. Patient is in a supine position with his face turned in such a way that the MSP is rotated at 45 degrees from the X-ray film.
3. Infraorbitomeatal line is perpendicular to the plane of the film.
4. CR is directed at an angle of 10 degree caudad.
5. CR enters 2.5 cm anterior and 1.9 cm above the external auditory canal (EAC).

Modified Chausse III View

1. Modified Chausse III view was defined by Czerny et al[3] and is a variation of the Stenvers view.
2. The modified Chausse III projection is obtained with the patient's back to the table.
3. The head is rotated 30 degrees (from the midline) away from the side to be imaged, and the CR X-ray beam is angled 15 degrees cephalad (above the Frankfurt plane).
4. This view produces less overlap of deeply inserted electrode arrays than the Stenvers view and projects the point of electrode insertion inferior to the vestibule.

Transorbital View

1. The transorbital view is a frontal view of the mastoid and petrous pyramid.
2. It can be anteroposterior or posteroanterior view.
3. The posteroanterior projection is obtained when the patient is facing the film with the chin flexed so that the orbitomeatal line is perpendicular to the tabletop.
4. The anteroposterior projection is obtained with the patient's back to the table with the chin flexed such that the orbitomeatal line is perpendicular to the tabletop.
5. The central beam is directed toward the center of the orbits, perpendicular to the detector.
6. The transorbital view nicely demonstrates the full length of the internal auditory canal, as well as the cochlea, vestibule, and SCCs.
7. The transorbital view can also be used in assessment of electrode position, especially in cases of bilateral CI. The main drawback in this view is that the depth of insertion cannot be assessed.

Towne's View

1. Dr E.B. Towne of England in 1926 described Towne's view.
2. Patient is positioned with the nuchal ridge placed against the image detector.
3. It is an anteroposterior view of the skull with 30 degree tilt from above and in front (**Fig. 6.4**).
4. The infraorbitomeatal line is perpendicular to the image receptor.
5. It shows both petrous pyramids, which can be compared and used in bilateral CI.
6. Both petrous pyramids of temporal bones, arcuate eminence, SSCC, mastoid antrum, internal acoustic canal, cochlea, EAC, dorsum sellae, foramen magnum, and posterior clinoid process can be visualized in this view.

Protocols for the postoperative imaging of CI vary among institutions, but most utilize either a variation of the Stenvers view or Transorbital view to visualize the electrode placement. In these views, normally inserted electrode arrays will follow a gentle curve in the first turn of the cochlea going into the second turn, with regular spacing between electrodes. Electrode array integrity and insertion depth can be reliably assessed using plain radiographs as long as the electrode array demonstrates a normal configuration. When an electrode array is compressed or bent, or has an atypical curvature, plain radiographs are not adequate to determine the location of the array. In these instances, a CT scan will generally be required.

It is difficult to have all children less than 3 to 4 years of age maintain the optimum positioning in the awake state, therefore 50/0 degree anteroposterior oblique projections, instead of a posteroanterior oblique view, are routinely performed on all young children just prior to extubation

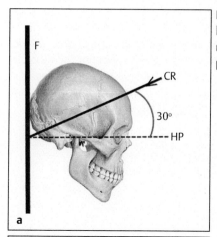

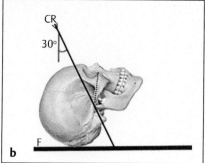

Fig. 6.4 (a, b) Towne's view with the head tilted by 30 degrees (CR, central ray, dotted black line; HP, horizontal plane; F, film).

intraoperatively, to document electrode position. In the anteroposterior projection the patient, during surgery, is in the supine position, and the head is turned away from the implanted side, similar to the posteroanterior projection, so that the MSP is again 50 degrees to the plane of the film and the central X-ray beam is parallel to the horizontal line. It should be noted that anteroposterior radiograph delivers a higher radiation dose to the lens of the eye which is considered radiosensitive. Using leaded glass or a small field of view can minimize potential injury to the lens. The best interobserver agreement about the depth of electrode insertion is achieved with the X-ray beam passing through the axis of the modiolus, which is perpendicular to the plane of the basal turn of the cochlea.[4]

Interpretations

A well-done X-ray mastoid (cochlear view) can show outline of various landmarks of inner ear such as middle ear, cochlea, round window, vestibule, and lateral and superior SCC with the electrode array (**Fig. 6.5**).

1. The vestibule (V) is identified as an oval lucency, which is directly lateral to the Internal acoustic canal (IAC).
2. Inferiorly, it is bordered by the most proximal extremity of the basal turn of the cochlea.

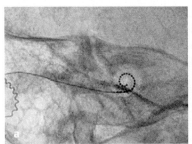
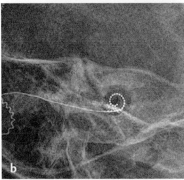
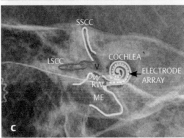

Fig. 6.5 (a, b, c) Postoperative X-ray modified Stenvers view showing intra-cochlear electrode array and various structures: SSCC, superior semicircular canal; LSCC, lateral semicircular canal; V, vestibule; OW, oval window; RW, round window; and ME, middle ear.

3. Superiorly, the SSC appears as a vertical lucent line or elliptical ring surrounded by the dense bony capsule.
4. The superior bony margin of the SSC forms a convexity on the roof of the petrous bone; this convexity is called the arcuate eminence.
5. Laterally, the LSCC is also seen as a horizontal lucent elliptical ring.
6. The bony capsule of the cochlea is visualized as an extremely dense shadow just at the bottom of the IAM.
7. The multichannel intracochlear electrode array appears as a two-dimensional spiral with its basal part located inferiorly.
8. The round window is not visualized on a plain radiograph but is indicated by the extension of the line drawn through the apex of the SSC and the midpoint of the vestibule reaching the electrode array.

There are various things which we can see with the help of a routine X-ray. These include:

1. Correct placement of electrode array.
2. Insertion depth.
3. Misplaced electrode array.
4. Kinking of electrode array: intra/extra cochlear.
5. Tip rollover.
6. Anterograde/retrograde electrode array insertion in case of a middle turn cochleostomy.
7. Position of receiver stimulator package.
8. Position of the magnet.

Correct Placement of Electrode Array

The aim of CI surgery is to insert the electrode array in the scala tympani of the basal turn and initial part of the middle turn of the cochlea, with least trauma to the cochlea and the electrode. It should be remembered that an electrode is replaceable but the cochlea is not. However, it should be understood that an electrode placed in a wrong manner or at the wrong place may affect the results for the whole life of the patient.

The qualities of a well-placed electrode array on radiograph include:

1. A fully inserted electrode array but not over inserted: This means all the electrodes are seen medial to the round window, inside the cochlea and at the same time, extra length of the electrode array is not inserted inside the cochlea (**Fig. 6.6**). The number of electrodes medial to the round window can be counted to confirm. This can be assessed with help of insertion depth also (discussed in the next section).
2. Equally spaced electrodes.
3. Wide arc subtended by the electrode array in the shape of the curve of the cochlear turns.
4. A gentle curve of the array in the cochlea, with no sharp turns or kinks.

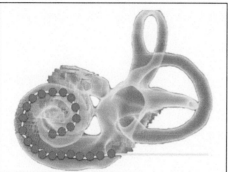

Fig. 6.6 Schematic representation of the correct placement of the electrode array (yellow color) and electrodes (blue color) seen medial to the round window.

Insertion Depth

The best way to calculate the depth of insertion of an electrode array is by measuring the angle of depth of insertion. Major work in this regard has been done by Cohen et al (1996), Marsh et al (1993), and Xu et al (2000).[1,2,5] This is done by drawing some lines on the radiograph. The first line is a vertical line drawn from the apex of the SSCC to the center of the vestibule. The point where this line intersects the shadow of the electrode array approximates the round window. The second reference line passes through the round window and the center of the spiral of the electrode array. This second line is the reference line for calculating angulation of the electrode insertion depth. The angle made by distal-most electrode with this 0 degree reference line is the insertion depth (**Fig. 6.7**). The angular depth of insertion varies between different types of electrode arrays. Med-El Ltd electrodes are usually longer and therefore have higher values as compared to Advanced Bionics Ltd and Cochlear Ltd electrodes. Authors consider that this value, depending on the type of electrode array, between 420 and 600 degrees is good for results.

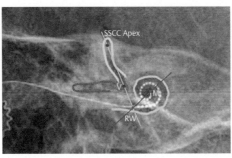

Fig. 6.7 Postoperative X-ray modified Stenvers view showing the method for estimating the depth of insertion. Geometric construction involves drawing a reference line through the apex of the superior semicircular canal (SSCC) and the midpoint of the vestibule (V) estimating round window (RW) and entry of the electrode array (light blue line) and then constructing a line perpendicular to the reference line passing through the electrode array spiral center (red line). A third line is drawn from the center of the electrode array spiral to the distal most electrode (yellow line). The angle between the red and yellow line with an additional 360 degrees, if needed, is the angular depth of insertion.

Number of Electrodes Inserted

Both partial and over insertion are bad for the outcomes. While partial insertion of electrode array will lead to lesser stimulation (**Fig. 6.8a–c**), over insertion (**Fig. 6.9**) will lead to missing out on basal turn spiral ganglion cells and possible inner ear trauma. The number of electrode shadows medial to the promontory or the round window can be counted to ascertain this. Various models of various companies have different numbers of electrodes, markers, and stiffening rings which need to be considered while counting the electrodes. Number of active intracochlear electrodes in Advanced Bionics Ltd is 16 (**Fig. 6.8d**), in Cochlear Ltd is 22 (**Fig. 6.8e** and **f**), and in Med-El Ltd is 12 (**Fig. 6.8g**). There are 10 stiffening rings proximal to the active electrodes in the REST model of Cochlear Ltd which are seen just like electrodes in radiograph. Other models of every company have markers which may or may not be seen on radiograph.

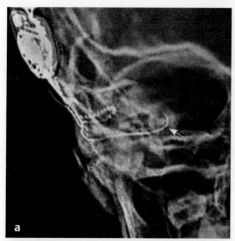

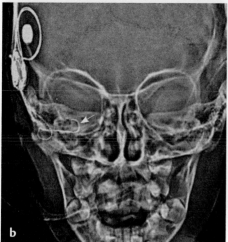

Fig. 6.8 (a, b) Postoperative X-ray transorbital view showing partial insertion of the electrode array, with a yellow arrow pointing toward the partially inserted electrode array. *(Continued)*

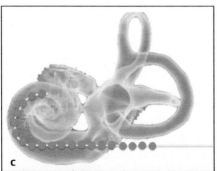

Fig. 6.8 *(Continued)* **(c)** Schematic representation of partial insertion of the electrode array (yellow color) with electrode (blue color). Postoperative X-ray modified Stenvers view showing normal electrode insertion of various available companies. **(d)** Advanced Bionics Ltd, **(e)** Cochlear Ltd 632 model, **(f)** Cochlear REST model with 10 proximal stiffening rings. *(Continued)*

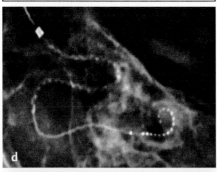

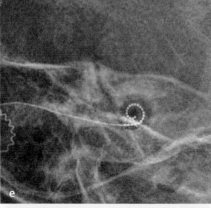

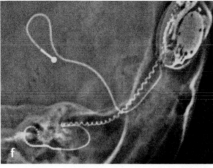

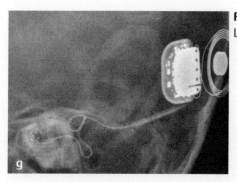

Fig. 6.8 *(Continued)* **(g)** Med-El Ltd.

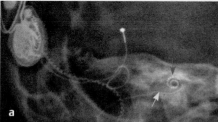

Fig. 6.9 **(a)** Postoperative X-ray modified Stenvers view showing over insertion of the electrode array, with yellow arrow pointing toward the round window and red arrow toward starting of the active electrodes. **(b)** Schematic representation of over inserted intracochlear electrode array (yellow color) with electrode (blue color).

Misplaced Electrode Array

Complex middle ear anatomy and its variations have led to quite a few misplaced electrodes arrays. The arrays have been put in hypotympanic cells, vestibule, SCCs, internal acoustic canal, carotid canal, eustachian tube, etc.[6] Intraoperative X-ray would help in diagnosing these misplaced arrays and correcting them before finishing the surgery. This would prevent the patient from undergoing a revision surgery. Whenever the gentle curve of the electrode array corresponding to cochlear turns is not seen, a misplaced array should be suspected **(Fig. 6.10)**. However, it should be remembered that sometimes even when the curve is seen, the array may not be in the

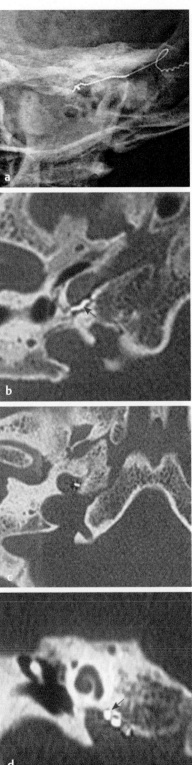

Fig. 6.10 **(a, b, c)** Showing a misplaced electrode array (blue arrow) into the internal carotid artery (red arrow). **(a)** Postoperative X-ray Modified Stenvers view showing loss of gentle curvature of the electrode array, thereby indicating a possibility of misplaced electrode array. **(b, c)** HRCT temporal bone axial view of the same patient confirming that the electrode array has actually got misplaced into the carotid canal. **(d)** HRCT temporal bone coronal view demonstrating the same.

right position, for example, in vestibular/SCC insertion, more so when modiolus hugging electrodes are being used, as the electrode gets curved due to its own memory. In such cases, a properly taken X-ray, in the right orientation plays an important role. Intraoperative CT scan can be done if available to confirm. If detected intraoperatively, a reinsertion can be tried with change in axis of insertion. If a misplaced electrode array is diagnosed/ suspected in the postoperative period then a follow-up CT should be done to see the exact positioning of the electrode array and to find out the reasons for this error (**Figs. 6.10, 6.11, 6.12, 6.13,** and **6.14**). A revision surgery would then be needed which may require a new implant in many cases.

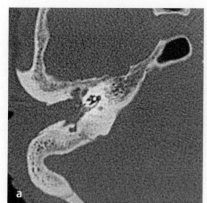

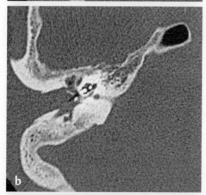

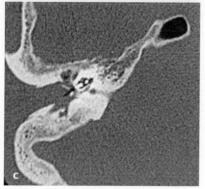

Fig. 6.11 (a, b, c) Postoperative CT after middle turn insertion in the revision surgery after the case shown in **Fig. 6.9**. Middle turn insertion was required in this case as the basal turn had been meddled during the previous surgery and was found to be ossified and lumen could not be found.

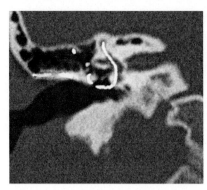

Fig. 6.12 Postoperative HRCT temporal bone coronal section bone window showing misplaced electrode array going into the superior semicircular canal, which required a revision surgery.

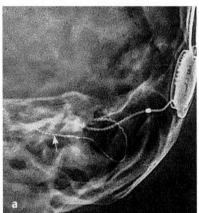

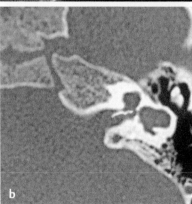

Fig. 6.13 **(a)** Postoperative X-ray modified Stenvers view showing misplaced electrode array (yellow arrow) in the internal acoustic canal. **(b)** HRCT temporal bone axial view showing the same in a malformed cochlea: SMS CVM type IIIb (incomplete partition 1).

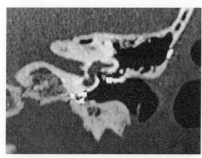

Fig. 6.14 HRCT temporal bone coronal sections showing pink arrow pointing toward the misplaced electrode array in the hypotympanum. This can happen more often in a well-pneumatized temporal bone and a well-developed subcochlear canaliculus.

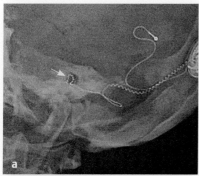

Fig. 6.15 Case of common cavity malformation with inserted electrode array. **(a)** Postoperative X-ray modified Stenvers view showing yellow arrow pointing to the electrode array inserted in a case of common cavity malformation. **(b)** Postoperative HRCT temporal bone axial view demonstrating the same.

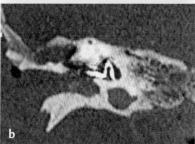

Insertion in Cases of Cochlear Malformations

One of the most interesting things to see is the technique of electrode insertion in a common cavity through the transmastoid labyrinthotomy (as we read in chapter on "Inner ear malformations"). The radiograph shown is no less interesting to see the U-shaped full banded electrode array inserted in a patient with common cavity deformity, such that the electrodes are in contact with the lateral wall where the nerve endings are present (**Fig 6.15**).

Tip Rollover

Rarely during insertion of the electrode array, the tip of the array may fold over itself (**Fig. 6.16**). Majority of studies mention 1 to 2% incidence; however, some studies mention up to 7% of tip foldovers in their series.[7] Few studies have found associations with right-sided CI, perimodiolar electrodes (4.7 vs 0.8%)[7] and round window insertions. Tip foldover may be missed if we rely completely on electrophysiological measurements. Impedances and neural responses obtained can be normal (sometimes, short circuits may be shown in nearby electrodes). To find out tip rollover, the audiologist will need to do SOE (spread of excitation) and EFI (electric field imaging) testing. However, these are advanced tests and are not done as a routine in all surgeries. If tip rollover is detected intraoperatively (by radiology or SOE/EFI), the surgeon may decide to reinsert the electrodes. If detected on postoperative radiology, observation and follow-up or selective deactivation of overlapping electrodes or revision surgery may be planned.

Kinking

If an electrode array is forced inside the cochlea against resistance or in a wrong direction, the electrode array may get kinked (**Fig. 6.17**). This may happen inside or outside the cochlea.

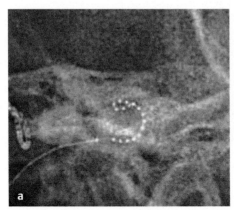

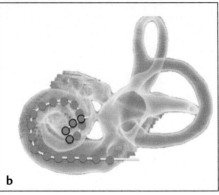

Fig. 6.16 **(a)** Postoperative X-ray modified Stenvers view showing tip rollover of the electrode array. **(b)** Schematic representation of tip rollover of the electrode array (yellow color) with electrode (blue color). The distal most four electrodes in A and B are showing the tip roll over.

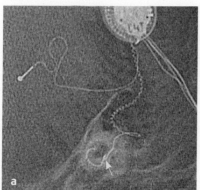

Fig. 6.17 **(a, d, e)** Postoperative X-ray modified Stenvers view, **(b)** HRCT temporal bone, oblique sagittal reconstruction image, **(c, f)** Schematic representation of the kinking of the electrode array. *(Continued)*

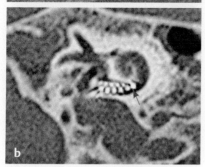

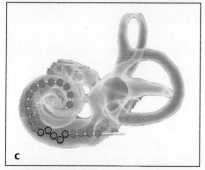

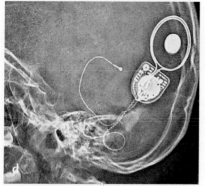

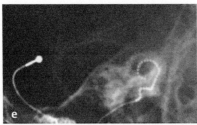

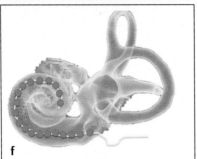

Fig. 6.17 *(Continued)* **(a, d, e)** Postoperative X-ray modified Stenvers view, **(b)** HRCT temporal bone, oblique sagittal reconstruction image, **(c, f)** Schematic representation of the kinking of the electrode array.

Magnet Displacement

Sometimes, due to trauma any time after surgery, the magnet of the implant may slip out of its socket. This may lead to pain and difficulty in attaching the external unit. Different views like skull anteroposterior view, lateral view, and cochlear view show that the magnet is not in the center of the coil but displaced toward the periphery (**Fig. 6.18**).

Cochlear Stenting

Sometimes, arranging the funds for cochlear implantation may need some time. This may specially be detrimental in cases of labyrinthitis ossificans due to progressive ossification. Kirtane et al described use of depth gauge (insertion test device), as an off-label use, for stenting the cochlear lumen to prevent further ossification and keeping a lumen patent for an electrode array to go in.[8] **Fig. 6.19** showed one of the patients who had significant ossification in basal turn and therefore middle turn cochleostomy was done and depth gauge was left inside. After 4 months, a formal CI surgery was done where depth gauge was removed and electrode array of CI was inserted. It is important that depth gauge and electrode array should be of same model.

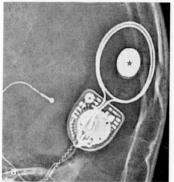
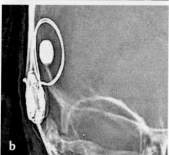
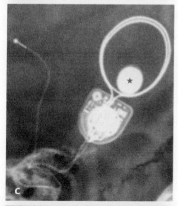
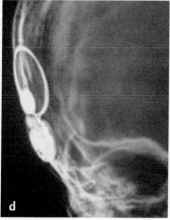

Fig. 6.18 (a, b, c, d) Postoperative X-ray modified Stenvers view and Towne's view: **(a, b)** Magnet (red asterisk) in normal position. **(c, d)** Magnet (red asterisk) misplaced inferiorly after trauma.

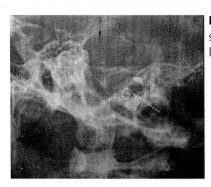

Fig. 6.19 Postoperative X-ray showing stenting with a depth gauge in a case of labyrinthitis ossificans.

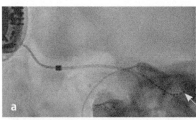

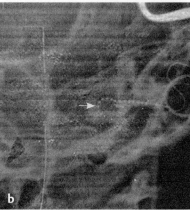

Fig. 6.20 Intraoperative X-ray modified Stenvers view showing **(a)** antegrade electrode array insertion (yellow arrow), and **(b)** retrograde electrode array insertion (yellow arrow) via middle turn cochleostomy in a case of labyrinthitis ossificans.

Middle Turn Insertions

In cases of ossified cochlea (as we read in the previous chapter), we may need to perform middle turn cochleostomy in certain conditions. Intraoperative radiograph or C-arm image becomes imperative in such cases. This is important not only to see correct placement of the electrode array but also to see whether the insertion has been antegrade toward the apical turn or retrograde toward the basal turn. Normally, we see that the curve of the electrode array is directed superiorly. It is also the same in antegrade insertions **(Fig. 6.20a)** after middle turn cochleostomy; however, in retrograde insertions the turn of the electrode array is seen to be directed inferiorly **(Fig. 6.20b)**. This is important to realize, as postoperative mapping by the audiologist will have to be reversed for retrograde insertions.

Electrode Extrusion

If there is intraoperative damage to the EAC, the electrode array with time can get extruded into the canal (**Fig. 6.21**). Electrode array in such a condition will come to lie in the EAC and epithelium can grow inside the mastoid antrum from the canal leading to iatrogenic cholesteatoma.

Can MRI be Done after Cochlear Implantation?

MRI compatibility of CIs is progressively getting better. Till a few years back, we only had MRI compatibility up to 1.5 T and that also needed magnet removal. Now the majority of patients with CIs can undergo 1.5-T MRI without magnet removal and advanced implants can even get up to 3.0-T MRI. However, the artifact of magnet may not allow that side of the brain to be visualized (**Fig. 6.22**). If a patient is expected to get an MRI of the ipsilateral brain (e.g., patients with acoustic neuroma) in future, then the option of magnet removal in the implant will be more beneficial.

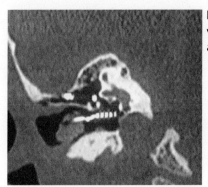

Fig. 6.21 HRCT temporal bone coronal view showing an extruded electrode array in external auditory canal.

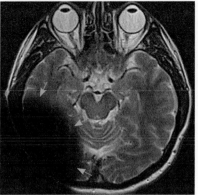

Fig. 6.22 MRI Brain with CI showing artifact (blue arrows) due to magnet in the CI in situ on the right side.

References

1. Marsh MA, Xu J, Blamey PJ, et al. Radiologic evaluation of multichannel intracochlear implant insertion depth. Am J Otol 1993;14(4):386–391
2. Xu J, Xu SA, Cohen LT, Clark GM. Cochlear view: postoperative radiography for cochlear implantation. Am J Otol 2000;21(1):49–56
3. Czerny C, Steiner E, Gstoettner W, Baumgartner WD, Imhof H. Postoperative radiographic assessment of the Combi 40 cochlear implant. AJR Am J Roentgenol 1997;169(6):1689–1694
4. Todd NW, Ball TI. Interobserver agreement of coiling of Med-El cochlear implant: plain X-ray studies. Otol Neurotol 2004;25(3):271–274
5. Cohen LT, Busby PA, Whitford LA, Clark GM. Cochlear implant place psychophysics 1. Pitch estimation with deeply inserted electrodes. Audiol Neurotol 1996;1(5):265–277
6. Ying YL, Lin JW, Oghalai JS, Williamson RA. Cochlear implant electrode misplacement: incidence, evaluation, and management. Laryngoscope 2013;123(3):757–766
7. Dhanasingh A, Jolly C. Review on cochlear implant electrode array tip fold-over and scalar deviation. J Otol 2019;14(3):94–100
8. Kirtane MV, More YI, Mankekar G. Cochlear stenting: how I do it. Eur Arch Otorhinolaryngol 2010;267(6):985–987

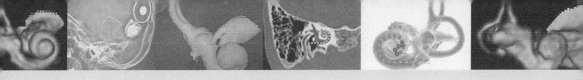

Chapter 7

Recent Advances

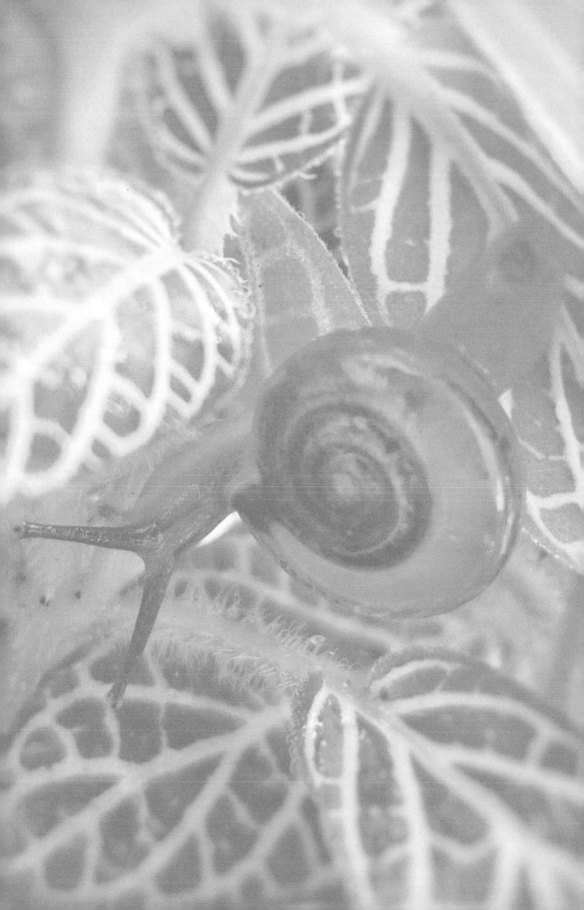

7 Recent Advances

Introduction

Cochlear implant (CI) surgery involves dealing with young children and intricate microscopic anatomy. Advances in radiology have helped in predicting many intraoperative issues and preventing complications. Few such advances are now being commonly used in many centers, a few are used in special circumstances and a few are in research phase. In this chapter, we will be reading about such advances in radiology which have made lives of surgeons easier and the surgery safer. These include:

1. C-arm fluoroscopy.
2. Cone-beam computed tomography (CBCT).
3. Navigation based/computer-assisted cochlear implant surgery.
4. Diffusion tensor imaging (DTI) and fiber tractography (FT).
5. Single-photon emission CT (SPECT)/positron emission tomography.
6. Functional magnetic resonance imaging (MRI).

In this chapter, author intends to discuss these one by one.

C-arm Fluoroscopy

The name C-arm is derived from the C-shaped arm used to connect the X-ray source and X-ray detector to one another (**Fig. 7.1**). Its special semicircular design allows the physician to move it more freely, covering the patient's whole body and taking images wherever needed. C-arms have radiographic capabilities, though they are used primarily for fluoroscopic intraoperative imaging during orthopedic procedures. It has found use in various types of implants. In CIs, it is commonly used to do "check" intraoperative X-ray imaging to confirm correct placement of the electrode array and implant, which has been discussed in earlier chapters. It gives faster and better images than the conventional portable X-ray machines. It gives high-resolution X-ray images in real time, thus allowing the physician to monitor progress and immediately make any corrections.

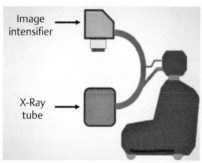

Fig. 7.1 Line diagram of C-arm machine which includes X-ray tube and an image intensifier. X-ray tube emits X-rays that penetrate the patient to produce an image that is captured by the image intensifier and is displayed on the monitor.

The C-arm machine is an X-ray image intensifier too. It converts X-rays into clear visible light better than the ordinary fluorescent screens. With this intensifying effect, low-intensity X-rays are seen in a brighter manner, helping the surgeons to view the X-rayed object more clearly. The C-arm machine is a fluoroscopy system too. Fluoroscopy is a technology which provides real-time X-ray imaging. It is particularly useful for guiding various diagnostic and interventional procedures. During CI surgery in cases with normal anatomy, an intraoperative plain film radiograph is sufficient to confirm the electrode position. Intraoperative fluoroscopy is indicated in cases with severely malformed inner ears where there is an increased chance of extracochlear electrode array placement and array insertion into the internal acoustic canal (IAC), as in SMS CVM type IIIb or IP3/IP1. These are typically those malformations where lamina cribrosa is deficient/absent leading to a wide communication between cochlea and IAC. Since the C-arm fluoroscopy technology enables the machine to provide real-time, high-resolution X-ray images, the surgeon can monitor the progress of the procedure and make decisions accordingly.

Fluoroscopy can be of two types:

1. Continuous fluoroscopy: It involves viewing live images (not acquiring images).
2. Pulsed fluoroscopy: It involves viewing intermittent live images to reduce dose during long procedures.

Pulsed fluoroscopy is preferred as it reduces the radiation exposure to the human lens. The dose of radiation produced by most modern units is below 10 rads per minute of use. The total exposure of radiation should be kept below 200 rads and the exposure time should not be more than a total of 1 to 3 minutes of short multiple exposures for CI. This can be used to generate static digital images or dynamic digital videos of electrode insertion.

Technique

The patient is placed in a supine position on the table with the head turned away from the operating surgeon. The C-arm with the beam generator is placed beneath the table directed in an anti-Stenvers view (in contrast to traditional Stenvers view, where the ear of concern is placed against the image plate). This not only magnifies the image of the cochlea by narrowing and centering of the beam but also minimizes the radiation exposure to the patient (**Fig. 7.2**).

Advantages

With the help of intraoperative fluoroscopy, insertional trauma to neuroepithelial elements and delicate inner ear structures can be minimized. Insertion endpoint can be precisely defined using fluoroscopy, thereby avoiding both electrode and structural damage. Excessive pressure application during electrode insertion should be avoided. The biggest advantage is early detection and correction of electrode arrays that get misplaced into the internal acoustic meatus.

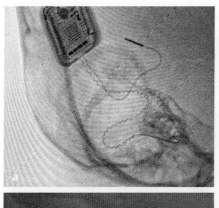

Fig. 7.2 **(a, b)** Intraoperative fluoroscopy images showing correct placement of intracochlear electrode array.

Cone-Beam Computed Tomography

Imaging after insertion in CI is important intraoperatively or postoperatively whether it is radiography, fluoroscopy, or high-resolution CT (HRCT) to confirm the correct placement of the electrode array. The major limitations of plain radiography and fluoroscopy are their poor image resolution of the intracochlear structures and the lack of a three-dimensional (3D) view thus sometimes missing to detect the misplacement of electrode arrays. HRCT temporal bone provides better resolution with sagittal, axial, and coronal views; however, the platform is fixed, and hence imaging cannot be performed intraoperatively. CBCT, however, has a mobile platform and can be used intraoperatively if needed. Also, CBCT gives higher spatial resolution and dynamic range; it has shorter acquisition and rapid scanning time, has less intense metallic artifacts, and lower radiation exposure than conventional multislice HRCT. As mentioned in the previous chapters, CBCT was primarily developed for dental and maxillofacial imaging and is now used in CI.

Technique

CBCT uses a rotating gantry on which an X-ray tube (source) and detector are attached (**Fig. 7.3**). A cone-shaped X-ray beam is directed through the middle of the temporal bone onto a two-dimensional X-ray detector. In contrast to conventional CT, which uses a narrow fan-shaped beam

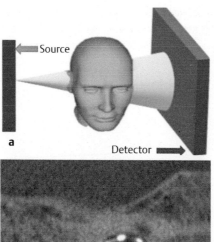

Fig. 7.3 **(a)** Schematic representation of cone-shaped CBCT. **(b)** Intraoperative CBCT showing normally inserted electrode array into the scala tympani of the cochlea.

requiring multiple rotations around the patient to create a volume of data, CBCT requires only a single rotation of a cone-shaped beam. The resolution of CBCT is usually between 75 and 300 Km which determines the size of the voxels and produces reconstructed images in the three orthogonal planes. Intraoperative CBCT is ideal in cases of inner ear malformations and pathological narrowing of the intracochlear lumen as in labyrinthitis ossificans where there is an increased risk of electrode array misplacement or tip rollovers. It provides reliable image quality for eliminating misplacement of electrode arrays into the vestibule or semicircular canals or foldover of the inserted array; for measuring the insertion depth angle and length of insertion; and for counting the number of electrodes inserted, which makes it a practical radiologic technique for assessment of electrode array positioning in the operating room (**Fig. 7.3**).

Role of Navigation in Cochlear Implantation

The results of cochlear implantation have improved with time by adapting newer and better technology. The better understanding of inner ear deformities and their physiology has led to improved outcomes. This in turn has expanded the indications for implantation and also surgical expertise required for managing such complex deformities. The use of navigation systems in complex cases would definitely be of immense help to the surgeon.

Navigation system has become a standard requirement for endoscopic sinus surgery as it helps in preventing complications and improves outcomes. Similar benefit has not been replicated in lateral skull base surgery due to lack of submillimeter accuracy. Also, the requirement for reviewing a side screen during an important step makes it difficult for the surgeons. The lack of any feedback, like audio feedback with facial nerve monitor further makes it less friendly to use. Thus, the need for intraoperative C-arm, X-ray has increased to localize and confirm the correct position of the electrode. The use of intraoperative CT scan and 3D volume tomography or rotational tomography has further improved the accuracy of electrode localization on table.[1,2]

A good navigation system should have good accurate registration with minimal invasion (**Fig. 7.4**). This will aid in more accurate localization. The traditional systems with less than 2 mm error have been useful in drill out procedures and while using split array electrode insertion in far advanced otosclerosis.[3] The use of anatomical landmarks and surface attached, or preferably implanted markers help in better anatomical localization.[3]

The use of navigation system is of paramount importance in minimally invasive robotic cochlear implantation. It helps identify, based on trajectory, a safe (>0.4 mm) and unsafe (<0.1 mm) distance from the facial nerve.[4] The reliability of navigation based robotic cochlear implantation is well described in literature.[5] The use of feedback through addition of neural electromyography (EMG) monitoring along with navigation has further improved the surgeon's comfort levels.[4] The integration of the navigation system and EMG monitoring helps in gaining feedback and the surgeon then does not have to shift his vision. The same can also be utilized in nonrobotic surgeries of complex inner ear malformations. The compound action potential measurements and intraoperative radiology though good, are not totally foolproof and thus a real time navigation will be of immense support to attain the best possible outcomes.[1]

Diffusion Tensor Imaging and Fiber Tractography

Various researches are going on in the field of radiology to assess the central auditory pathway. Peter Basser introduced the DTI technique in 1994.[6] It is done with the help of conventional MR machines. DTI data is acquired using a single-shot, spin-echo, echo-planar imaging sequence. DTI data of fractional anisotropy (FA) is used to assess changes in tissue density, damage to myelin sheath and white matter. Therefore in patients with peripheral hearing loss, the central auditory pathway undergoes changes, which are picked up by DTI. FT is 3D reconstruction of the data collected by DTI to assess the neural tracts. It follows color codes (**Fig. 7.5**):

- Transverse fibers: red.
- Anteroposterior fibers: green.
- Craniocaudal fibers: blue.
- Oblique fibers: as per the color originating along the direction of obliquity.

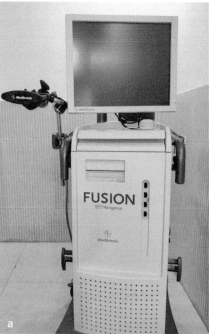

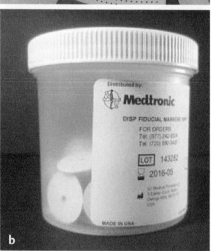

Fig. 7.4 **(a)** The navigation system used by the authors for skull base surgery. **(b)** The fiducial surface markers are placed preoperatively and CT scan is obtained. They are left in place and utilized for registration intraoperatively for better anatomical localization.

Study by Chang et al[7] found that good outcome cochlear implant patients had higher FA values in several brain areas, including Broca's area, genu of corpus callosum and auditory tract. Similarly, study by Huang et al[8] found that in poor outcome patients, there are reductions in FA values at trapezoid body, superior olivary nucleus, inferior colliculus, medial geniculate body, auditory radiation, and white matter of Heschl's gyrus. However, the practical usability of these modalities still needs to be proved.

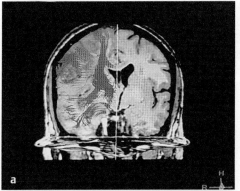

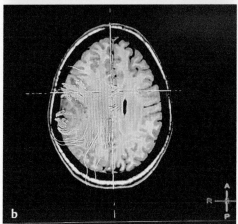

Fig. 7.5 (a, b) Diffusion tensor imaging and fiber tractography images showing neural tracts in brain.

Single-Photon Emission Computed Tomography/Positron Emission Tomography

Duration of auditory deprivation is considered as one of the principal indicators to predict the outcomes of hearing and speech perception after CI. Long-standing prolonged sensorineural hearing loss (SNHL) causes neural degeneration of the spiral ganglions and atrophy of the cochlear nuclei and thus showing less benefit post CI when compared to individuals with a brief history of auditory deprivation. Several neuroimaging modalities have been used for presurgical evaluation to predict outcomes of CI. Techniques such as PET and SPECT can be used to detect cortical responses to auditory and speech stimuli in individuals planned for cochlear implantation or using CIs. PET assesses the rate of metabolism and SPECT assesses the regional cerebral blood flow in the auditory cortex in response to auditory stimuli. SPECT recognizes several activation patterns in the cerebral cortex in response to different stimuli. SPECT mainly uses radioisotope tracers such as 99mtechnetium-hexamethylpropyleneamine oxime (99mTc-HMPAO).[9]

A bilateral, simultaneous acoustic stimulus, consisting of pure multi-frequency tones (250 Hz, 500 Hz, 1000 Hz, 2000 Hz, and 4000 Hz), at the highest available intensity (125 dB-HL) is presented through headphones to detect responses in the auditory cortex. Studies indicate that the overall resting metabolism of persons with long-standing deafness differs from normal-hearing individuals. Individuals who are deaf demonstrate a reduction in the cortical responses to acoustic inputs in the region of primary auditory cortex (Brodmann Areas 41, 42) and auditory association cortices (Brodmann Areas 21, 22, and 38). SPECT imaging may help in determining the better ear for implantation preoperatively by revealing the strongest, most intact pathway activated during auditory stimulation when all routine audiometric findings are equal across both ears. Studies also suggest a strong relationship between the level of speech perception performance achieved with cochlear implantation and the activation patterns associated with primary auditory and auditory association cortices.[9,10,11]

Functional MRI

Functional MRI (fMRI) is a neuroimaging modality that makes use of blood oxygenation level dependent (BOLD) contrast to measure the changes in the brain activity based on the changes in blood flow that occur during neuronal activation. In relation to CIs, fMRI can be used to assess the residual hearing function in the primary auditory cortex region and also can be used as a prognostic neuroimaging biomarker to predict speech perception and language outcomes after cochlear implantation. It is usually done under sedation in children and an auditory narrow band noise or chirp stimulus with a threshold above 90 dB is presented. Cortical activation following auditory stimulus results in localized increase in blood flow which results in a change in signal intensity in MRI (**Fig. 7.6**). The activated and nonactivated regions in the cortex have different signal intensities, and brain activation maps can be attained. Studies have shown a positive correlation, that is, activity in the temporo-parieto-occipital junction, areas in the prefrontal cortex, and the cingulate gyrus before implantation have better outcomes in speech and language function post implantation.[12,13]

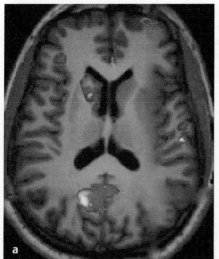
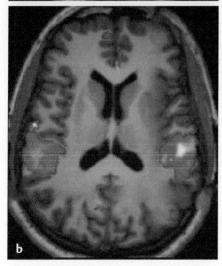

Fig. 7.6 fMRI images of the auditory cortex area in response to auditory stimulus in subjects **(a)** with profound hearing loss and **(b)** with normal hearing.

Conclusion

Radiology has always been of help in predicting the outcomes of various surgeries, including CIs. With these advances, the surgeons will be able to predict outcomes in a better way and prevent complications. One of the major advances being the ability to assess the central auditory pathway, which till now has been evaluated only to a limited extent. Also, intraoperative use of radiology has progressed from a basic X-ray to the use of navigation making the surgical mishaps negligible.

References

1. Kim CS, Maxfield AZ, Foyt D, Rapoport RJ. Utility of intraoperative computed tomography for cochlear implantation in patients with difficult anatomy. Cochlear Implants Int 2018;19(3):170–179

2. Aschendorff A, Maier W, Jaekel K, et al. Radiologically assisted navigation in cochlear implantation for X-linked deafness malformation. Cochlear Implants Int 2009;10(Suppl 1):14–18

3. Dejaco D, Prejban D, Fischer N, et al. Successful cochlear implantation of a split electrode array in a patient with far-advanced otosclerosis assisted by electromagnetic navigation: a case report. Otol Neurotol 2018;39(7):e532–e537

4. Ansó J, Scheidegger O, Wimmer W, et al. Neuromonitoring during robotic cochlear implantation: initial clinical experience. Ann Biomed Eng 2018;46(10):1568–1581

5. Bell B, Gerber N, Williamson T, et al. In vitro accuracy evaluation of image-guided robot system for direct cochlear access. Otol Neurotol 2013;34(7):1284–1290

6. Basser PJ, Mattiello J, LeBihan D. MR diffusion tensor spectroscopy and imaging. Biophys J 1994;66(1):259–267

7. Chang Y, Lee HR, Paik JS, Lee KY, Lee SH. Voxel-wise analysis of diffusion tensor imaging for clinical outcome of cochlear implantation: retrospective study. Clin Exp Otorhinolaryngol 2012; **5**(1, Suppl 1)S37–S42

8. Huang L, Zheng W, Wu C, et al. Diffusion tensor imaging of the auditory neural pathway for clinical outcome of cochlear implantation in pediatric congenital sensorineural hearing loss patients. PLoS ONE 2015;10(10):e0140643. Published 2015 Oct 20.

9. Di Nardo W, Giannantonio S, Di Giuda D, De Corso E, Schinaia L, Paludetti G. Role of auditory brain function assessment by SPECT in cochlear implant side selection. Acta Otorhinolaryngol Ital 2013;33(1):23–28

10. Suárez H, Mut F, Lago G, et al. Changes in the cerebral blood flow in postlingual cochlear implant users. Acta Otolaryngol 1999;119(2):239–243

11. Allen A, Barnes A, Singh RS, Patterson J, Hadley DM, Wyper D. Perfusion SPECT in cochlear implantation and promontory stimulation. Nucl Med Commun 2004;25(5):521–525

12. Deshpande AK, Tan L, Lu LJ, Altaye M, Holland SK. fMRI as a preimplant objective tool to predict children's postimplant auditory and language outcomes as measured by parental observations. J Am Acad Audiol 2018;29(5):389–404

13. Deshpande AK, Tan L, Lu LJ, Altaye M, Holland SK. fMRI as a preimplant objective tool to predict postimplant oral language outcomes in children with cochlear implants. Ear Hear 2016;37(4):e263–e272

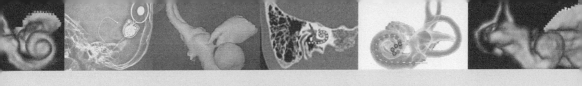

Chapter 8

Preoperative Checklist Prior to Cochlear Implantation

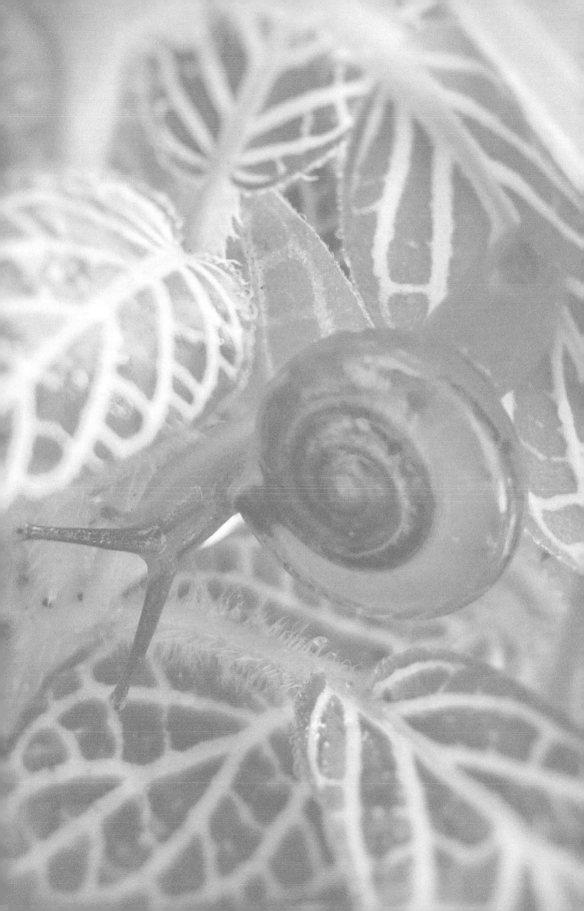

8 Preoperative Checklist Prior to Cochlear Implantation

Introduction

As we discussed in the first chapter, cochlear implantation is about teamwork and the communication between a radiologist and a surgeon is of paramount importance. Candidacy, surgery, complications, and prognosis can all be decided based on radiology of that individual patient. With advances in radiology and implants, these things would keep on increasing.

In this chapter, author presents a checklist of computed tomography (CT) and magnetic resonance imaging (MRI) which can be used while reporting the scans. This may be changed from institute to institute depending on the facilities available and the team involved.

Checklist

Name of the patient:

Age:

Sex:

Date of imaging:

Apart from the above basic information, **Tables 8.1** and **8.2** provide checklists for high-resolution CT (HRCT) and MRI of temporal bones respectively.

Table 8.1   Checklist for HRCT temporal bones

Variable	Right	Left
Skull thickness		
Mastoid pneumatization (Hyperpneumatized/sclerotic/normal)		
Otic capsule		
Pinna/external auditory canal anomalies		
Korner's septum		
Middle ear cleft • Aerated/soft tissue density/any other thing		
Ossicles • Malleus • Incus • Stapes		
Facial nerve • Anomalous course or dehiscent		
Sigmoid sinus		
Tegmen plate		
Jugular bulb		
Internal carotid artery		
Hypotympanum		
Subcochlear canaliculus		
Facial recess		
Cochlea • Number of turns • Modiolus • Cochlear aperture • Interscalar septum • Patency of cochlea • Lamina cribrosa • Orientation of cochlea • Cochlear duct length • Malformation, if any		
Vestibule		
Semicircular canals		
Vestibular aqueduct		
Cochlear aqueduct		
Internal acoustic meatus		

Abbreviation: HRCT, high-resolution computed tomography.

Table 8.2 Checklist for MRI brain and temporal bones

Variable	Right	Left
Middle ear cleft		
Cochlea • Number of turns • Modiolus • Cochlear aperture • Interscalar septum • Patency/fluid signal of cochlea • Malformation, if any		
Internal acoustic canal		
Cochlear nerve		
Vestibule		
Semicircular canals		
Endolymphatic duct and sac		
Vestibular aqueduct		
Cochlear aqueduct		
Cerebellopontine angle		
Brainstem		
Brain		
Any other significant anomaly		
Previous ear surgery status		

Abbreviation: MRI, magnetic resonance imaging.

Index